W0106188

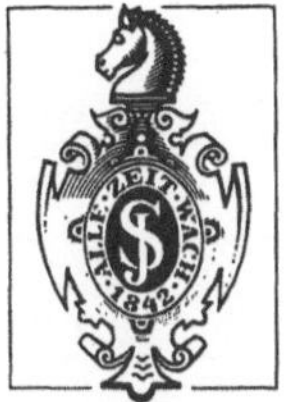

D. R. Krishna U. Klotz

Clinical Pharmacokinetics

A Short Introduction

With 26 Figures
and 18 Tables

Springer-Verlag
Berlin Heidelberg New York
London Paris Tokyo
Hong Kong Barcelona

Dr. Devarakonda Rama Krishna
College of Pharmaceutical Sciences, Kakatiya University
Warangal 506 009, India

Professor Dr. Ulrich Klotz
Dr. Margarete Fischer-Bosch-Institut
für Klinische Pharmakologie
Auerbachstraße 112, D-7000 Stuttgart 50
Federal Republic of Germany

Translation
of "Ulrich Klotz, Einführung in die Pharmakokinetik"
Govi-Verlag, Frankfurt/Main, Federal Republic of Germany
ISBN-13:978-3-540-52458-8

ISBN-13:978-3-540-52458-8 e-ISBN-13:978-3-642-75623-8
DOI: 10.1007/978-3-642-75623-8

Library of Congress Cataloging-in-Publication Data
Krishna, D. R. (Devarakonda Rama)
Clinical pharmacokinetics: a short introduction / D. R. Krishna. U. Klotz. p. cm.
Rev. translation of: Einführung in die Pharmakokinetik / Ulrich Klotz.
ISBN-13:978-3-540-52458-8
1. Pharmacokinetics. I. Klotz, Ulrich, 1943- . II. Klotz, Ulrich, 1943- Einführung in die Pharmakokinetik. English. III. Title.
[DNLM: 1. Pharmacokinetics. QV 38 K92p] RM301.5.K75 1990 615'.7—dc20 DNLM/DLC for Library of Congress 90-10067 CIP

2129/3145-543210 Printed on acid-free paper

Contents

Part I

Basic pharmacokinetics

Historical note

"Pharmacokinetics" is a relatively new field and its development to the present status took less than 100 years. Some important mile stones in its progress are

1910 – Bateman ("Bateman function")
1927 – Widmark (estimation of alcohol in blood)
1932 – Widmark (elimination of alcohol and acetone)
1937 – Teorell (kinetics of distribution and introduction of compartment model)
1949 – Druckrey and Küpfmüller (a book entitled "Dose and Action")
1953 – Dost (a book entitled "Der Blutspiegel"). The term "pharmacokinetics" was first coined.
1960 – Garrett (analog computer)
– E. Krieger-Thiemer (drug dosage)
1961 – Dettli (simulation of plasma concentration-data). The term "biopharmaceutics" was introduced.
1962 – First Congress of Pharmacokinetics was held in Germany.
– *Since then:* development of different computer programmes for pharmacokinetic analysis (e.g. SAAM, NONLIN, PROPHET, MULTI, RIP).

Today, with the help of computers it is possible to fit plasma concentration-time data to an appropriate pharmacokinetic model to estimate different parameters. Mathematical and statistical equations have been developed to individualize the dosage regimen of drugs which may often pose problems during therapy. Programs such as MAXSIM will enable one to simulate plasma and tissue concentration-time profiles based on cmpartmental or perfusion model parameters.

1 Introduction and definitions

The understanding of pharmaco-kinetic and -dynamic properties of a drug is essential for rational approach of the treatment. In addition, knowledge of pharmacokinetics is particularly important to make the therapy more effective and safe.

Pharmacokinetics, which essentially deals with the mathematical definition of movement of drug (in and out of body), helps in understanding and assessing the pharmacodynamic response. With the knowledge of pharmacokinetics one can easily explain terms like onset, duration and intensity of drug action (therapeutic as well as toxic). The change in concentration of drug and its metabolite(s) with respect to time in plasma and tissues can even explain different underlying (patho-) physiological changes in the body.

1.1 Mathematical basics

The mathematical expressions which are useful for determination of different pharmacokinetic parameters are discussed in the following section.

1.1.1 Linear pharmacokinetics

As the name implies, there exists a linear relationship between the dose D administered and the concentration C in blood or plasma or serum ($C \sim D$). The decline in concentration (elimination) of the drug and its metabolites takes place according to 1st order kinetics. Therefore, the rate of change in concentration, dc/dt is proportional to the concentration C of the drug in blood

$$dc/dt \sim C \quad \text{or} \quad dc/dt = -k \cdot C \tag{1}$$

where k is the proportionality constant; also known as the elimination rate constant.

Through integration and rearrangement we get the exponential form

$$C(t) = C(0) \cdot e^{-k \cdot t} = C(0) \cdot 10^{-k \cdot t/2.303} \tag{2}$$

where C(0) and C(t) are the plasma concentrations at time 0 and t respectively.

The elimination rate constant can be obtained from the slope of semi-logarithmic plot of concentration-time data and the plasma half-life ($t_{1/2}$) is calculated using the following equation

$$t_{1/2} = 0.693/k \tag{3}$$

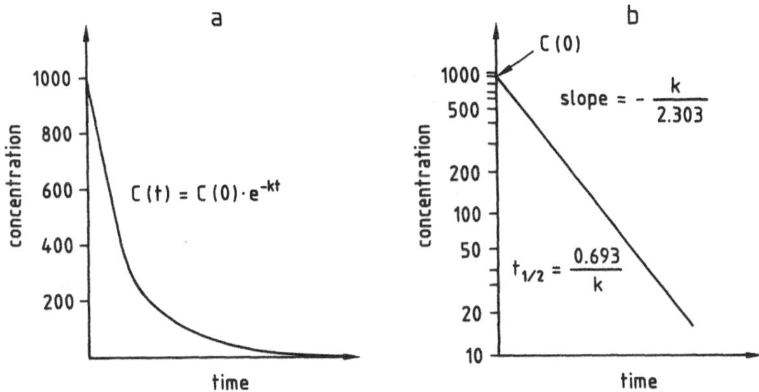

Fig. 1 a, b. Schematic representation of 1st order rate process. **a** Exponential fall in plasma concentration with time following i.v. administration, when plotted on arithmatic graph paper. **b** Same data, showing a linear relation, plotted on a semi-log graph paper; a straight line with slope $= -k/2.303$ and y-axis intercept C(0). The elimination half-life can be calculated from the equation $t_{1/2} = 0.693/k$

The fall in drug concentration following intravenous administration is exponential when plotted on an arithmatic graph paper and it becomes linear when plotted on a "semi-log" paper (Fig. 1). It implies that the drug is eliminated according to first order kinetics preceded by a rapid distribution in the body. In such a situation it may be assumed that the entire body represents a single and homogenous unit. Calculation of important pharamcokinetic parameters (by graphical approach) of a drug, which confers 1-compartment model characteristics on body, following i.v. administration is explained here with an example.

Model problem 1

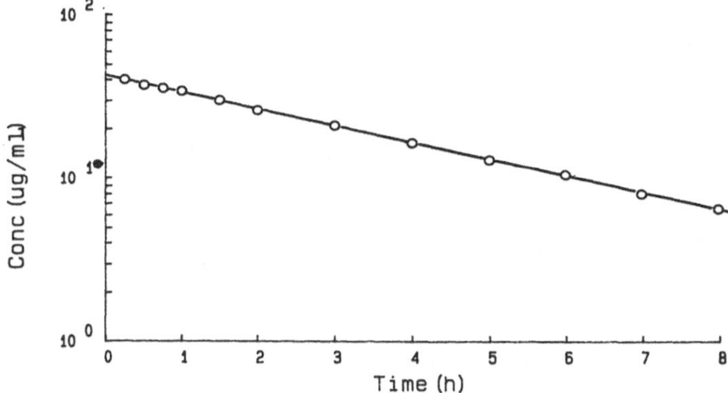

The table below gives the plasma levels of a new drug, which is under clinical trial in a healthy subject (weighing 70 kg) following 500 mg i.v. administration.

Plot the data on a semi-logarithmic graph paper (time on linear X-axis and concentration on logarithmic Y-axis). Assuming that the kinetics of the drug are best explained by 1-compartment open model, estimate

(1) Initial plasma concentration, C(0)
(2) elimination rate constant, k and
(2) half-life, $t_{1/2}$ (also read $t_{1/2}$ directly from the graph).

Time (h)	Conc. (μg/mL)	Time (h)	Conc. (μg/mL)
0.25	40	3.00	21
0.50	37	4.00	16.5
0.75	35.5	5.00	13
1.00	34	6.00	10.5
1.50	30	7.00	8.00
2.00	26	8.00	6.50

Solution:

(1) initial concentration (Y-axis intercept), C(0) = 42 μg/mL.
(2) −Slope = [log(20) − log(10)]/2.9
Slope = 0.104
$k = -2.303 \times \text{Slope} = 0.24\ h^{-1}$
(3) terminal half-life, $t_{1/2} = 0.693/k = 2.9$ h.

Distribution and elimination of many drugs can be characterized by using this model, the so called "one compartment open model" (schematically shown in Fig. 2a). For some drugs, however, elimination shows a bi-exponential behaviour (Fig. 2) because of two distinct and simultaneous processes. Following i.v. administration one may notice an initial, rapid distribution phase ("α-phase") followed by a slower elimination phase ("β-phase"). When the body exhibits heterogenity with respect to distribution of a drug thereby showing a biphasic fall, we assume that it represents not one, but two units or compartments, hence the expression "two compartment open model". By definition it should be possible to determine "half-life" of the drug during these two phases with the help of the equations

$$t_{1/2(\alpha)} = t_{1/2\,\lambda_1} = 0.693/\lambda_1 \quad (3a)$$

$$t_{1/2} = t_{1/2\,\lambda_z} = 0.693/\lambda_z \quad (3b)$$

where λ_1 and λ_z are called disposition constants and are not to be interchanged with k.

In case of extravascular administration, absorption must take place prior to distribution and elimination. The plasma concentration profile depicts two opposite and simultaneous processes namely absorption (invasion) and elim-

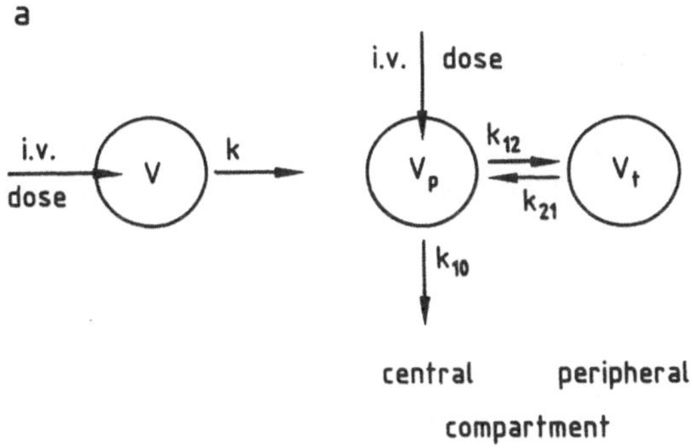

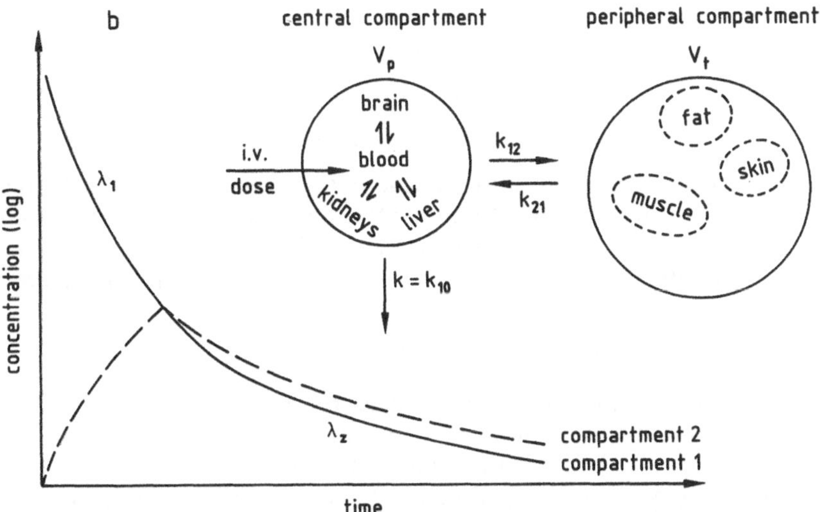

Fig. 2a, b. Schematic representation of different compartment models with corresponding distribution volume terms and rate constants. **a** 1-compartment open model, which represents the body as a single distribution compartment with volume V. **b** 2-compartment open model, the body is represented on the basis of differences in perfusion as two compartments, central ($V_p = V_c$) and peripheral (V_t). The rate constants k_{12} and k_{21} describe the drug transfer between the two compartments and the elimination rate constant k or k_{10} characterizes the elimination process from the central compartment. λ_1 and λ_z are the disposition constants corresponding to rapid distribution phase and slower elimination phase

ination (evasion). If X is the amount of drug remaining at the site of absorption

$$dX/dt \sim X \quad \text{or} \quad dX/dt = -k_a \cdot X \tag{4}$$

where k_a is the absorption rate constant.

At time $=0$, the amount of drug available at the site of absorption X(0) is identical to the dose D administered. Therefore

$$X = X(0) \cdot e^{-k_a \cdot t} = D \cdot e^{-k_a \cdot t} \tag{5}$$

If A is the amount of drug absorbed until time t in the body

$$A = D - X = D - D \cdot e^{-k_a \cdot t} = D(1 - e^{-k_a \cdot t}) \quad (6)$$

As the concentration is proportional to the amount, the above equation may be written in terms of concentration by using volume of distribution V (see also page 33).

$$C \sim A \quad \text{or} \quad C = A/V \quad (7)$$

$$C(t) = D/V \cdot (1 - e^{-k_a \cdot t}) \quad (7a)$$

As elimination also takes place simultaneously the rate equation is expressed as difference between these two rate processes

$$dA/dt = k_a \cdot X - k \cdot A \quad (8)$$

$$= k_a \cdot D \cdot e^{-k_a \cdot t} - k \cdot A \quad (9)$$

Solving this differential equation and rewriting it in terms of concentration results in the equation (10) developed by Bateman (Bateman's function)

$$C(t) = F \cdot (D/V) \cdot [(k_a/(k_a - k))\,(e^{-k \cdot t} - e^{-k_a \cdot t})] \quad (10)$$

and this form is applicable only in case of 1-compartment open model. In addition to absorption and elimination reversible distribution also takes place simultaneously between blood and tissues. At a given time, if A_p and A_t represent the amounts of drug in blood (plasma) and tissue compartments respectively then equation (8) becomes

$$dA/dt = k_a \cdot X - k_{10} \cdot A_p - k_{12} \cdot A_p + k_{12} \cdot A_t \quad (11)$$

where k_{12} and k_{21} are first order rate constants for the distribution process and k_{10} is the apparent elimination rate constant.

The drug may also be measured in urine to compute the kinetic parameters. From the amount of unchanged drug excreted in urine (Ae) up to the time points t and infinity (∞), it is possible to determine the elimination rate ("Sigma-Minus method"). Half-life can be calculated using k (see also page 24).

Besides half-life, there is another important parameter called "area under plasma concentration-time curve (AUC)", which is extremely useful to differentiate linear and non-linear kinetics. There are several methods of estimating this parameter including

(1) cut and weigh
(2) trapezoidal rule and
(3) planimetry.

Among these three, trapezoidal rule is most popular. The concentration-time curve is divided into different segments (each of them is a trapezoid) and the area of each segment is computed using area equation of a trapezoid (Fig. 3). Summation of individual areas yields AUC(0 − t). The extrapolated area from time t to infinity (∞) is obtained from the formula

$$AUC(0 - t) = ((t_{i+1} - t_i)/2) \cdot (C(i) + C(i+1)) \quad (12)$$

$$AUC(t - \infty) = C(\text{last})/\lambda_z\,. \quad (12a)$$

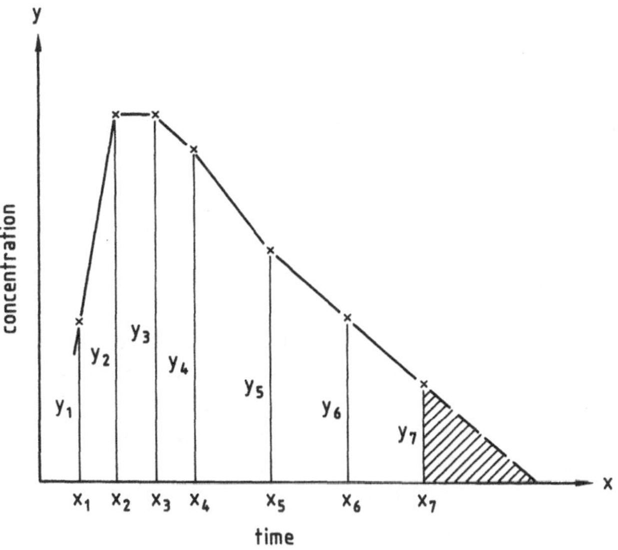

Fig. 3. Application of trapezoidal rule: The area under each segment is calculated first and the total area upto the last measured concentration is then obtained by summation of individual areas. The area upto infinity is calculated by using the equation (12a)

The equation for the total area is given as

$$\mathrm{AUC}(0-\infty)=\int_0^\infty \mathrm{C}\cdot \mathrm{dt}=\mathrm{AUC}(0-\infty)+\mathrm{C(last)}/\lambda_z\,. \tag{13}$$

One can also compute AUC$(0-\infty)$ using the points of intersection on the ordinate and disposition constants. A general form is given below

$$\mathrm{AUC}=\mathrm{C}_1/\lambda_1+\mathrm{C}_2/\lambda_2+\ \dots\ +\mathrm{C}_n/\lambda_n \tag{14}$$

where n is the number of compartments.

In case of linear kinetics, AUC analogous to plasma concentrations is proportional to the administered dose. For example, doubling the dose will increase the AUC by a factor 2.

Model problem 2

Using the data of model problem 1 and the trapezoidal rule, estimate

(1) AUC$(0-t)$

(2) AUC$(t-\infty)$ and

(3) AUC$(0-\infty)$.

Solution:

(1) $AUC(0-t) = (0.5) \cdot (0.25) \cdot (42+40) + (0.5) \cdot (0.25) \cdot (40+37)$
$+ (0.5) \cdot (0.25) \cdot (37+35.5) + \ldots$
$= 152.9\ \mu g \cdot h/mL.$

(2) $AUC(t-\infty) = 27.1\ \mu g \cdot h/mL.$

(3) $AUC(0-\infty) = 179.98\ \mu g \cdot h/mL.$

1.1.2 Nonlinear pharmacokinetics

In certain exceptional situations, when the dose is increased beyond a particular amount (resulting near toxic levels in plasma), the kinetics may no longer be linear and plasma concentrations along with AUC will not be proportional to the administered dose. Elimination rate and half-life will also become dose and concentration dependent. Some drugs show this phenomenon of non-linearity following multiple and high dose administration.

Certain processes such as biotransformation, protein or tissue binding and biliary secretion require enzyme or carrier systems. These systems are specific and have only limited capacity for the substrate molecules. Presence of large excess of drug (substrate) at such a capacity limited system can lead to saturation of the available sites and may result in "non-linear kinetics".

Drugs like valproic acid, disopyramide and salicylic acid in concentrations above therapeutic level may lead to saturation of binding sites of plasma proteins resulting in elevated concentrations of free drug (unbound fraction f_u).

Metabolism in liver, which involves specific enzymes is one of the most important factors that contributes to nonlinear kinetics. These enzyme mediated, capacity limited processes can be best explained by Michaelis-Menten equation

$$v = dM/dt = V_{max} \cdot C/(K_m + C) \qquad (15)$$

where v = reaction velocity and v_{max} = maximum reaction velocity.

In a normal situation (linear kinetics), at any given time the plasma concentration C is very much less than the Michaelis-Menten constant $K_m (C \ll K_m)$ and the above expression is in the form

$$v = V_{max} \cdot C/K_m = k \cdot C \qquad (16)$$

where

$$k = V_{max}/K_m \qquad (16a)$$

which is comparable to the equation for a 1st order reaction, where the reaction velocity is proportional to the concentration. In case of a capacity-limited system, where the enzyme is saturated with the substrate $(C \gg K_m)$, the equation (16) changes to the form

$$v = V_{max} \cdot C/C = V_{max} \qquad (17)$$

indicating that the process then follows zero order kinetics. It is obvious that the reaction is no longer dependent on concentration and proceeds at constant and maximum velocity. The elimination kinetics of ethanol is one of classical examples for the above phenomenon. The enzyme, alcohol-dehydrogenase which is responsible for the biotransformation of alcohol into acetaldehyde works under saturating substrate concentration resulting in zero order kinetics.

In case of phenytoin, another model drug which exhibits non-linear kinetics, the steady state plasma concentrations are not proportionally increased by increase in dose (doubling the dose may result in 3 to 5 fold increase in concentrations). This explains clearly that increasing the dose of drugs like phenytoin well within the therapeutic range may lead to saturation of enzymes and thereby ensuing levels higher than those expected in plasma.

A similar observation is made in case of salicylates, where a 50% increase in the maintenance dose may result in about 3 fold increase in plasma levels. Here, in addition to enzyme saturability another factor, limited availability of the conjugate (glucuronic acid) required for the formation of metabolite, is responsible for the reduced elimination. For both drugs an increase in dose (or plasma concentrations) results in the reduction of elimination rate. The half-life of salicylic acid is about 2 to 3 h following administration of doses smaller than 3 g and about 15 to 30 h following doses larger than 3 g.

1.2 Pharmacokinetic models

The approach of compartment models is useful for better understanding and proper interpretation of the concentration-time data. Body represents a system of different compartments with respect to the drug disposition though in reality these compartments have no anatomical or physiological existence. Pharmacokinetic analysis or characterization based on this concept enables prediction of plasma concentrations and subsequently the dosage regimen of the drug. The hypothetical compartmental approach is essentially based on distribution and elimination of the drug following absorption. These models are often called "open" (e.g. 1-compartment-open model) as the drug being a foreign substance, which ultimately eliminated from the body either in unchanged form or in the form of metabolite(s). The mass or material transfer into, out of and between different compartments takes place according to 1st order kinetics and each process is characterized by a specific rate constant. The compartmental analysis was first applied to plasma data in 1937 by Teorell. 1-compartment open model is simplest of all according to which the body represents a single and homogenous unit. Following intravenous administration, the drug is very rapidly mixed and diluted in the circulating blood. Then it is distributed throughout the body very quickly. Although the body is assumed to represent a single compartment, it does not mean that the drug concentration in all tissues and body fluids is the same or equal to the concentration in plasma. One may merely assume that the rate of change of concentration at these sites is comparable or proportionale to that in plasma. The concentration, however, is dependent on the dose administered and volume of distribution (see Fig. 1).

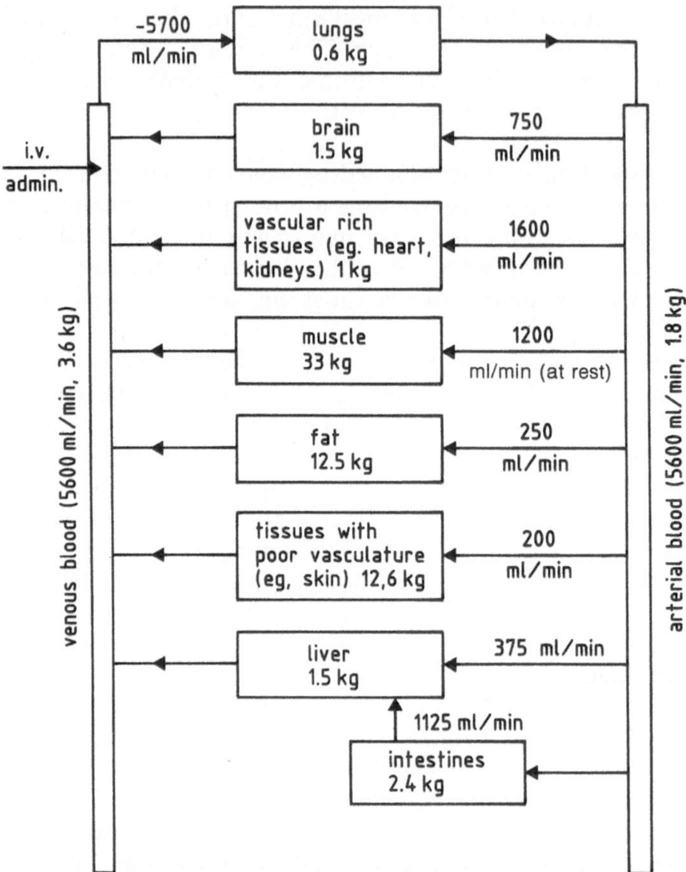

Fig. 4. The physiological perfusion model, which describes the distribution and elimination processes of an intravenously administered drug into different tissues or organs which exhibit differences in blood flow and mass

Pharmacokinetics of most drugs is better explained or characterized by the two compartment open model. The scheme and physiological background are shown in Figs. 2 and 4. Following i.v. administration the drug is mixed rapidly and distributed quickly to some tissues which are well perfused. The extent of penetration into tissues is dependent on the permeability of tissue membranes, tissue mass and solubility of the drug in tissue fluid. The postulation that there exists two compartments is perhaps an oversimplification, because the distribution of drug into various tissues in reality is more complex than one could imagine.

Blood and highly perfused organs (tissues) such as brain, heart, liver and kidneys together represent the "central compartment" (volume V_p or V_c). These tissues, due to better perfusion reach equilibrium very rapidly. On the other hand, poorly perfused tissues such as skin, skeletal muscle and fat together represent the "peripheral or tissue compartment" (volume V_t). In tissues, the drug levels first gradually increase, reach a peak and then decline even after i.v. administration (see Fig. 2).

It is possible to determine different rate constants for a drug administered intravenously, whose kinetics are best described by a two compartment model, using the method of residuals. Application of different equations for computation of some important parameters is explained in model problem 3.

The plasma concentration of drug which confers two compartment model characteristics of the body, at any given time t may be determined by the following biexponential equation

$$C(t) = C_1 \cdot e^{-\lambda_1 \cdot t} + C_z \cdot e^{-\lambda_z \cdot t} \quad (18)$$

where λ_1 and λ_z are apparent 1st order disposition constants (hybrid rate constants) and C_1 and C_z are zero time intercepts of residual and terminal lines on Y-axis, respectively.

Model problem 3

Plasma concentrations of famotidine (a H_2-receptor antagonist) following 20 mg i.v. administration, in a patient (weighing 65 kg) of reflux oesophagitis are given in the table below. Plot the data on a semi-log paper. Assuming that the drug confers 2-compartment model characteristics on the body estimate

(1) $\lambda_1, \lambda_2, C_1, C_z$

(2) $t_{1/2}(\lambda_1), t_{1/2}(\lambda_z)$

(3) k_{10}, k_{12}, k_{21}

(4) AUC

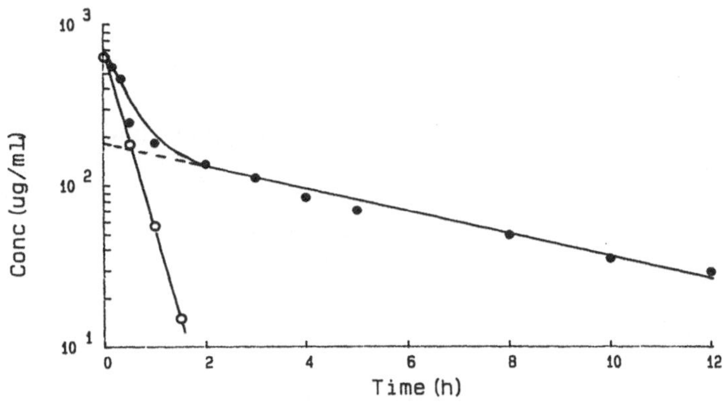

Time (h)	Conc (ng/mL)	Time (h)	Conc (ng/mL)
0.165	545.1	3.00	110.9
0.33	458.4	4.00	84.0
0.50	244.7	5.00	69.7
1.00	183.2	8.00	49.1
2.00	135.0	10.00	35.0
		12.00	29.0

Solution:

- Slope of residual line $=(\log(630)-\log(52))/1=1.08$

$$\lambda_1=1.08\times 2.303$$

$$\lambda_1=2.49\ \mathrm{h}^{-1}$$

$$t_{1/2}(\lambda_1)=0.693/\lambda_1=0.28\ \mathrm{h}$$

- Slope of terminal line $=(\log(54)-\log(37))/3$

$$\lambda_2=0.055\times 2.303$$

$$\lambda_2=0.126\ \mathrm{h}^{-1}$$

$$t_{1/2}(\lambda_z)=0.693/\lambda_z=5.5\ \mathrm{h}.$$

$$k_{21}=(\lambda_1\cdot C_z+\lambda_z\cdot C_1)/(C_1+C_z)$$

$$=0.59\ \mathrm{h}^{-1}$$

$$k_{10}=\lambda_1\cdot\lambda_2/k_{21}$$

$$=0.53\ \mathrm{h}^{-1}$$

$$k_{12}=\lambda_1+\lambda_z-k_{21}-k_{10}$$

$$=1.24\ \mathrm{h}^{-1}$$

$$\mathrm{AUC}=1122.3+230$$

$$=1352.5\ \mathrm{ng}\cdot\mathrm{h/mL}.$$

Method of residuals

This method is also described by terms like "stripping" and "feathering". It is a simple and convenient method, used for resolving a biexponential curve. In the present case, figure (3) depicts the distribution and elimination phases when the plasma concentrations are plotted against time on a semi-logarithmic paper.

As $\lambda_1>\lambda_z$, the term $C_1\cdot e^{-\lambda_1\cdot t}$ approaches zero earlier than the term $C_z\cdot e^{-z\cdot t}$ and the above equation becomes

$$C(t)=C_z\cdot e^{-\lambda_z\cdot t} \tag{19}$$

writing in common logarithms yields

$$\log C(t) = \log C_z - \lambda_z \cdot t/2.303 \quad (20)$$

which is the equation for the terminal phase of the curve with slope $= -\lambda_z/2.303$. The zero time intercept of this line is $\log C_z$. The difference between the measured concentration values during the distribution phase and the values corresponding to the extrapolated terminal phase yields a series of residual values. The residual concentration $C(r)$ is given by

$$C(r) = C_1 \cdot e^{-\lambda_z \cdot t} \quad (21)$$

writing in common logarithms yields

$$\log C(r) = \log C_1 - \lambda_1 \cdot t/2.303 \quad (22)$$

which is the equation for the residual line. The slope of this line $(-\lambda_1/2.303)$, gives the distribution rate constant and the zero time intercept yields $\log C_1$.

By using the following relationships, one can obtain different rate constants

$$\lambda_1 \cdot \lambda_z = k_{21} \cdot k_{10} \quad (23)$$

$$\lambda_1 + \lambda_z = k_{12} + k_{21} + k_{10} \quad (24)$$

$$k_{21} = (\lambda_1 \cdot C_z + \lambda_z \cdot C_1)/(C_1 + C_z) \quad (25)$$

$$k_{10} = \lambda_1 \cdot \lambda_z / k_{21} \quad (26)$$

$$k_{12} = \lambda_1 + \lambda_z - k_{21} - k_{10} \quad (27)$$

The logical continuation of this concept of "dividing the body into compartments" based on the difference in perfusion results in postulation of "multiple compartment models". It should be remembered that each compartment in such a model is kinetically homogenous. For example, in a three compartment open model, based on physiological basis one can hypothetically divide the body into (1) blood and organs with rich vasculature such as brain, heart, liver and kidneys (volume V_1), (2) muscle group (V_2) and (3) fat and the tissues with very poor vasculature (volume V_3).

In practice it is accurate enough if one computes the pharmacokinetic parameters assuming a "two compartment model", because the mathematical computation becomes more complex if the assumed number of compartments is too large. Plotting the plasma concentration-time data on a semi-logarithmic graph paper helps to predict the number of compartments. If the decline of plasma levels is mono-exponential (the data points lie on a single straight line), it implies that one compartment model is valid. Similarly a bi-exponential decline implies a two compartment model. Theoretically n-exponential decline implies an "n-compartment model". In practice, it is always desirable to have at least 4 measured data points in the tail portion of the curve for the estimation of terminal half-life as a model independent parameter by linear regression. If it is required to perform a multi-compartment analysis to investigate the polyexponential behaviour of drug disposition then measurement of the early plasma concentrations following i.v. administration is necessary.

The physiologic consideration of various distribution compartments is based on the difference in blood perfusion of different body regions. Figure 4 depicts some important details of various tissues including mass and blood flow. This perfusion model helps in predicting concentrations in different tissues depending on size and blood flow, provided that the experimentally determined tissue/plasma concentration ratio for the drug is known.

2 Absorption

Drug, administered by any route other than intravascular must be absorbed from the site of administration to reach blood circulation and has to cross many barriers (cell membranes) to reach the site of action (receptors). Different absorption sites which are of great importance include skin (percutaneous), skeletal muscle (intramuscular), respiratory tract (inhalation), mucous membrane of mouth (sublingual) and gastrointestinal tract (per oral and per rectum).

Despite large absorption area of 1.7 m^2, skin does not play a significant role in the absorption of drugs because of poor diffusion. However, it appears that there is a potential for the development of novel dosage forms such as transdermal drug delivery systems (e.g. skin plaster for nitrates and scopalamine), with the help of which it may be possible to maintain relatively constant plasma levels similar to i.v. infusion.

Respiratory tract with an absorption area of 70 m^2 is particularly suited for the administration of central depressants (e.g. general anaesthetics) and drugs which are poorly absorbed from g.i. tract (e.g. sodium chromoglycate) in aerosol form.

Administration of drugs through gastrointestinal tract offers several advantages like

(1) ease of administration (upto a few grams can be administered)
(2) largest absorption surface (about 120 m^2) and
(3) most drugs are taken orally (nearly 80%). A few are also administered rectally.

Although the cell structure of different absorption sites is morphologically different, the mechanism of absorption or transportation is more or less the same. The absorption membrane is a "protein-lipid-double layer" with distinct aqueous pores. Mechanisms of drug absorption and factors affecting absorption are briefly described in the following section.

2.1 Absorption mechanisms and physico-chemical factors

For absorption to take place, the administered dosage form (e.g. tablet or capsule) must undergo disintegration into fine particles followed by dissolution in the gastrointestinal fluids. Both solubility and absorption are dependent on various physicochemical properties including pKa or pKb and polarity of the drug.

Most of the drugs are chemically either weak acids or weak bases and the ionised and unionised forms of a drug exhibit great variation in their polarities. It is well known that the unionised form, which is more lipid soluble (with a high lipid/water partition coefficient) is better transported across the bilayer lipid membrane than its counter part.

Hydrogen ion concentration at the site of absorption can greatly influence dissolution and ionisation of the drug. It may be generalized that acidic drugs (e.g. phenytoin, phenobarbital, aspirin) are better absorbed in stomach as greater part of the drug remains unionised at acidic pH. On the other hand, basic drugs (e.g. amphetamine, quinine, morphine) are better absorbed in distal part of small intestine where the pH is alkaline. Acidic drugs are also well absorbed in intestines because of longer duration of stay and very large surface area of the intestinal mucosa.

Absorption of many drugs across the membrane takes place by a simple process of "passive diffusion". This process does not involve energy expenditure and the rate of diffusion is directly proportional to the concentration gradient across the membrane. The lipid soluble substances diffuse through the "fats" and the polar substances diffuse through the aqueous (hydrophilic) pores of the membrane. The aqueous pores with a diameter of about 30 Å allow only smaller molecules (MW < 60,000 D) to pass through.

Certain substances such as vitamins, amino acids and nucleic acids are transported by another mechanism known as "active diffusion", where the transportation takes place against concentration gradient and involves energy expenditure. This process usually takes place with the help of certain specific molecules known as "carriers" present in the membrane.

2.2 Physiological factors

In addition to physico-chemical and formulation factors some physiological factors also influence drug absorption. Bacteria of the intestinal flora for example synthesize enzymes like non-specific esterases which hydrolyse levo-dopa and different esters of penicillins (e.g. pivampicillin, talampicillin and carindacillin). As a result of this presystemic intestinal metabolism the amount of drug available for absorption is often significantly reduced. Blood perfusion at the site of absorption is also of great importance. For example, absorption of volatile anaesthetics through lungs is dependent on the pulmonary circulation. Similarly absorption of nutrients through gastrointestinal mucosa is influenced by the extent of perfusion. In case of congestive heart failure, perfusion is impaired due to reduction in cardiac output, which in turn can reduce the absorption of drugs (e.g. quinidine, procainamide, hydrochlorthiazide). Another major factor that may affect absorption of drugs is the gastric emptying rate, which is influenced by meal and drugs like atropine, metoclopramide and tricyclic antidepressants. Likewise the intestinal motility by affecting the time of contact of drug with the absorption surface may alter absorption.

The influence of these factors becomes more significant in case of poorly absorbed drugs. Absorption may be reduced in an increased gastrointestinal transit state such as diarrhoea or following administration of laxatives. In case of intramuscular or subcutaneous routes of administration the extent of circulation in the vicinity of "depot" plays a significant role. Absorption, following i.m. or s.c. administration can be improved by massage, fomentation and by administering drugs which enhance the local circulation. Similarly absorption can be reduced by administering vasoconstrictors like adrenaline.

2.3 Pharmacokinetic calculations

Following disintegration (e.g. tablet, capsule) and dissolution in the gastrointestinal fluids the drug is absorbed in most cases by simple diffusion. The plasma concentration-time curve is the result of these processes which take place simultaneously and it shows two phases, known as invasion and evasion phases respectively. During absorption phase (rising part of the curve) the rate of absorption is greater than the rate of elimination and during elimination phase (beyond the peak concentration) absorption ceases and only elimination occurs.

Peak concentration is higher and earlier following rapid absorption and it is lower and delayed following slower absorption. Poorly soluble drugs are incompletely absorbed and the absorption from solutions can be expected to be faster than from tablets and suspensions. Oxazepam has a more delayed onset of action than diazepam, because of its slower absorption due to its relatively high degree of polarity. This fact should be taken into consideration when it is indicated for induction of sleep.

For characterization of absorption and estimation of bioequivalence of different formulations of a drug, peak plasma concentration (C_{max}) and time taken for achieving the peak (t_{max}) are often taken into account. However, the extent and rate of absorption cannot exactly be assessed by these two parameters as two other processes, distribution and elimination are simultaneously taking place in addition to absorption (Fig. 5).

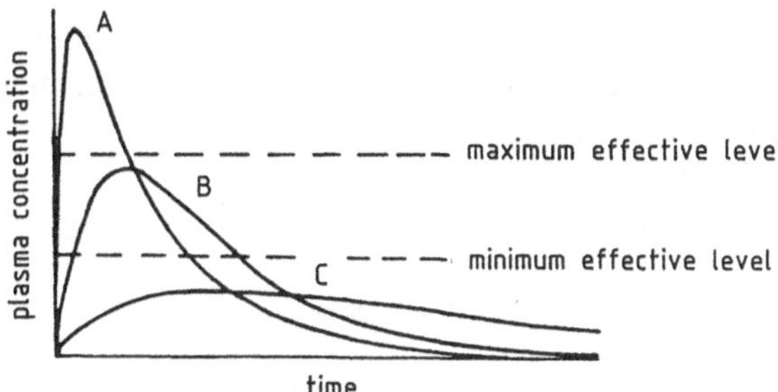

Fig. 5. Schematic representation of time-plasma concentration profiles following oral administration of a drug in different formulations *A* a solution, *B* a tablet or a capsule and *C* a depot preparation, depicting rapid, slow and very slow absorption processes. The concentrations should lie between the minimum and maximum levels to produce the therapeutic effect as seen in case of *B*. In case of *A* the concentrations are reaching toxic levels and in case of *C* the concentrations are in the ineffective range over the entire period of time

T_{max} is independent of pharmacokinetic model and dose of the administered drug. The exact time point at which peak occurs is difficult to be determined experimentally. However, it is possible to calculate this parameter by using the following equation

$$t_{max} = (1/(k_a - k)) \cdot \ln(k_a/k) = \ln(k_a/k)/(k_a - k) \quad (28)$$

Plasma peak concentration which is proportional to the dose administered can be calculated in case of one compartment model using the equation

$$C_{max} = (D/V) \cdot (k_a/k)^{k/(k-k_a)} \quad (29)$$

AUC is directly proportional to the amount of drug absorbed (see page 9). The delay in release of drug from a slow release dosage form (e.g. an enteric coated tablet) appears to be in agreement with the delay in appearance in blood. This delay, often called as "lag-time" depends primarily upon the gastric retention time. It represents the actual beginning of absorption. The equations for calculation of absorption kinetic parameters following administration of such formulation are derived taking the duration of availability of drug at the site of administration into account. Many formulations are developed based on these equations. However, in some occasions such as during the use of transdermal drug release systems and during altered physiological conditions, these equations need slight modifications.

Mathematically absorption can take place according to zero or 1st order kinetics. In the first instance absorption is analogous to intravenous infusion with a rate constant k_0. In most cases it is a first order process (see page 7) with a rate constant k_a.

There are different methods for the determination of absorption rate, which include

(1) method of residuals
  (a) from plasma concentration data and
  (b) from urinary excretion data (with some methodical prerequisites)
(2) Wagner-Nelson method (for one compartment model)
(3) Loo-Riegelman method (for multiple compartment models)
(4) deconvolution method (model independent)
(5) intercept method (model independent) and
(6) statistical moments method (model independent).

The first three methods are described here.

1. Method of residuals. This method, which has been discussed in the previous section for the resolution of i.v. bi-exponential curve can be also applied to plasma concentration data obtained following oral administration (with 1st order absorption). From equation (10), the plasma concentration of drug at any given time t, following administration of dose D, can be calculated provided the bioavailability F, is known. Assuming $k_a > k$, the term $e^{-k_a \cdot t}$ approaches zero and the equation (10; see page 8) becomes

$$C=(k_a \cdot F \cdot D/V(k_a-k)) \cdot e^{-k_a \cdot t} \tag{10a}$$

writing in logarithms

$$\log C=\log(k_a \cdot F \cdot D/V \cdot (k_a-k)-k \cdot t/2.303 \tag{10b}$$

Based on this equation, when the plasma concentrations following oral administration are plotted on a semi-logarithmic paper against time, a bi-exponential curve is obtained. Slope of the terminal linear phase ($-k/2.303$) which gives the elimination rate upon extrapolation to time zero yields an intercept equal to $\log(k_a \cdot F \cdot D/V \cdot (k_a-k))$. The concentration-time values in the absorption phase are subtracted from the values on the extrapolated line and the differences (residual concentrations) are then plotted against time. Slope of this new line ($-k_a/2.303$) gives the absorption rate (k_a).

Model problem 4

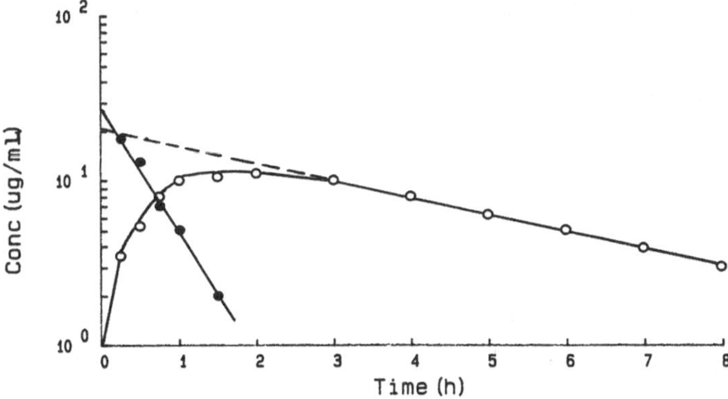

The following table gives the plasma concentrations of the same drug, which has been described in the model problem 1 in the same patient (weight, 70 kg) but following 500 mg p.o. administration.

Time (h)	Conc (μg/mL)	Time (h)	Conc (μg/mL)
0.25	3.5	3.0	10.0
0.50	5.3	4.0	8.0
0.75	8.0	5.0	6.2
1.0	10.0	6.0	5.0
1.5	10.5	7.0	3.9
2.0	11.0	8.0	3.0

Assuming 1st order absorption, estimate

(1) AUC, k, $t_{1/2}$
(2) t_{max}, C_{max} and
(3) k_a

Solution:

Elimination:

– Slope of terminal line = (log(8) – log(3))/4 = 0.107
$k = 0.107 \times 2.303 = 0.25\ h^{-1}$
$t_{1/2} = 0.693/0.25 = 2.77$ h

Absorption:

– Slope of residual line = (log(10) – log(5))/0.5 = 0.6
$k_a = 0.6 \times 2.303 = 1.38\ h^{-1}$
$t_{1/2\,(a)} = 0.693/1.38 = 0.5$ h

AUC = 56.05 + 12 = 68.8 µg · h/mL

$t_{max} = \text{In}(k_a/k)/(k_a - k)$
$= 1.71/1.13 = 1.51$ h

$C_{max} = (FD/V) \cdot e^{-k \cdot t_{max}}$
$= 0.4 \times 42 \times e^{-0.25 \times 1.51}$
$= 11.5$ µg/mL

This method can also be applied to urinary excretion data for the estimation of k_a. The urinary excretion of unchanged drug is given by the equation

$$A_e^{\infty} - A_e = (A_e^{\infty}/k_a - k)\,(k_a \cdot e^{-k \cdot t} - k \cdot e^{-k_a \cdot t}). \qquad (30)$$

As $k_a > k$, the term $k \cdot e^{-k_a \cdot t}$ approaches zero and the above equation becomes

$$A_e^{\infty} - A_e = (A_e^{\infty}/k_a - k) \cdot e^{-k \cdot t} \qquad (31)$$

writing in logarithms

$$\log(A_e^{\infty} - A_e) = \log(A_e^{\infty}/k_a - k) - k \cdot t/2.303 \qquad (32)$$

$(A_e^{\infty} - A_e)$ values are plotted against time and the slope of the terminal linear phase $(-k/2.303)$ gives the elimination rate. Subtracting the true $(A_e^{\infty} - A_e)$ values from the values on the extrapolated terminal phase yields the residuals $(A_e^{\infty} - A_e)$ which are plotted against time. The slope of residual line $(-k_a/2.303)$ gives absorption rate and the Y-intercept gives $(A_e^{\infty} \cdot k/k_a - k)$. An important prerequisite for this method is that many samples of urine at different time intervals (including at time = ∞) are to be collected after the administration of the drug.

Model problem 5

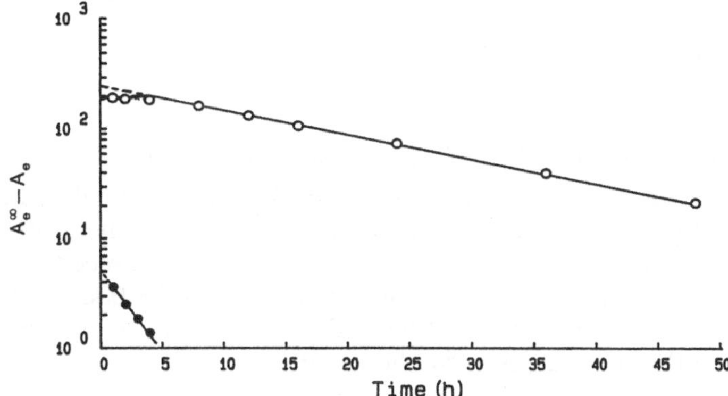

The following table gives the amount of an antibiotic excreted unchanged in the urine at different intervals of time (including at $t = \infty$; after 7 half-lives), of a patient (55 years) with a respiratory tract infection who received a single 300 mg oral dose. Assuming that the drug follows 1-compartment open model kinetics determine

(1) k, $t_{1/2}$

(2) k_a, $t_{1/2(a)}$

Time (h)	A_e (mg)	$A_e^\infty - A_e$
1	9.8	190.2
2	15.0	185.0
4	19.0	181.0
8	40.2	159.8
12	69.9	130.1
16	95.0	105.0
24	127.8	72.2
36	161.0	39.0
48	179.0	21.0
	200.0	–

Solution:

- Slope of terminal line $= (\log(130) - \log(72.2))/12 = 0.0213$

  $k \quad = 2.303 \times 0.0213$
  $\quad = 0.0491\ \text{h}^{-1}$

  $t_{1/2} \quad = 0.693/0.0491 = 14.1\ \text{h}$

– Slope of residual line $=(\log(50)-\log(14))/2=0.276$

$$k_a = 2.303 \times 0.276$$
$$= 0.635\ h^{-1}$$
$$t_{1/2\,(a)} = 0.693/0.635$$
$$= 1.1\ h.$$

2. Wagner-Nelson method. This method takes material balance equations of the absorbed drug into consideration. It has one advantage that it does not require i.v. data for the computations. However, it is applicable only for drugs which follow one compartment model kinetics. At any given instance following oral administration, if A_B is the amount of drug present in the body and A_{el} is the mount eliminated (through excretion and metabolism). The amount of drug absorbed till that time is given by the equation

$$A = A_B + A_{el} \tag{33}$$

Differentiation of the above equation with respect to time gives

$$dA/dt = dA_B/dt + dA_{el}/dt \tag{34}$$

It is known that

$$dA_{el}/dt = k \cdot A_B \tag{35}$$

substituting $k \cdot A_B$ for dA_{el}/dt in the equation (34) gives

$$dA/dt = dA_B/dt + k \cdot A_B \tag{36}$$

for a drug with one compartment model characteristics

$$dA/dt = V \cdot dC/dt + k \cdot V \cdot C \tag{37}$$

upon integration from time 0 to t and 0 to ∞, the above equation becomes

$$A(t) = V \cdot C(t) + k \cdot V \int_0^t C \cdot dt \tag{38}$$

and

$$A(\infty) = k \cdot V \int_0^\infty C \cdot dt \tag{39}$$

where $\int_0^t C \cdot dt$ and $\int_0^\infty C \cdot dt$ are AUCs upto time t and ∞ respectively.

From equations (38) and (39)

$$A(t)/A(\infty) = (C + k \int_0^t C \cdot dt)/k \int_0^\infty C \cdot dt \tag{40}$$

The above equation relates the cumulative amount of drug absorbed after a certain time to the amount of drug ultimately absorbed (fraction absorbed). A plot of percent unabsorbed $(100-(1-(A(t)/A(\infty))))$ versus time, if it yields a straight line on an arithmatic graph paper it suggests a zero order absorption (absorption rate $= -$slope). On the other hand, if it yields a straight line on a semi-log paper it suggests a 1st order absorption and the rate of absorption $= -2.303 \times$ slope).

Model problem 6

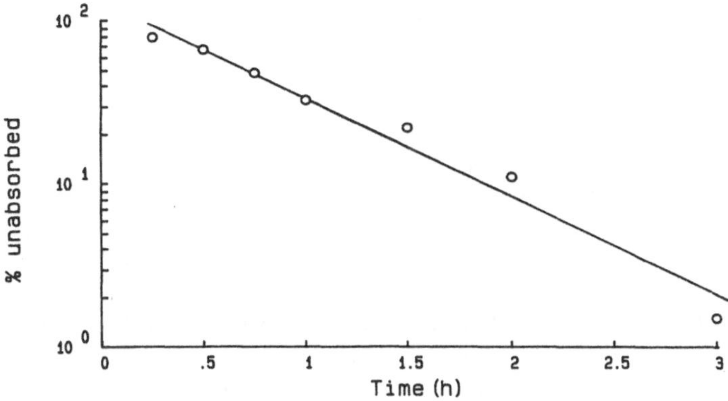

Estimate the absorption rate, k_a using the data of model problem 4, by Wagner Nelson method.

Solution:

Time (h)	Conc. (μg/mL)	AUC(0−t)	k × AUC	A(t)/V	[A(t)/A(∞)] × 100	% unabsorbed
0.25	3.5	0.44	0.11	3.61	21.0	79
0.5	5.3	1.54	0.39	5.69	33.7	66.3
0.75	8.0	3.20	0.80	8.80	52.2	47.8
1.00	10.0	5.45	1.36	11.36	67.4	32.6
1.50	10.5	10.58	2.65	13.15	78.0	22.0
2.00	11.0	15.95	3.99	14.99	88.9	22.0
3.0	10.0	26.45	6.61	16.61	98.5	11.1
4.00	8.0	35.45	8.86	16.86	100.0	1.5
5.00	6.2	42.55	10.63	16.83		
6.00	5.0	48.15	12.04	17.04		
7.00	3.9	52.60	13.15	17.05		
8.00	3.0	56.05	14.01	17.01		

Slope (as calculated by simple linear regression) is 0.504 and consequently $k_a = \text{slope} \times 2.303 = 1.16\ h^{-1}$.

3. Loo-Riegelman method. This method is applicable to linear multiple compartment models and requires both oral as well as i.v. data from the same subject. The mathematical equations may be derived as in the case of Wagner-Nelson method.

If A is the amount absorbed in the body, at any given time

$$A = A_p + A_t + A_{el} \tag{41}$$

where A_p and A_t are the amounts of drug present in plasma and tissue compartments respectively.

Differentiation of the above equation yields

$$dA/dt = dA_p/dt + dA_t/dt + dA_{el}/dt \tag{42}$$

by definition

$$dA_{el}/dt = k_{10} \cdot A_p \tag{43}$$

where k_{10} is apparent first order elimination rate constant.

The equation (42) may be written in terms of concentration and volume of distribution

$$(1/V_p) \cdot dA/dt = dC_p/dt + k_{10} \cdot C_p + (1/V_p) \cdot dA_t/dt \tag{44}$$

Integration of this equation between time limits $0-t$ and $0-\infty$ results in

$$A(t)/V_p = C(t)_p + k_{10} \int_0^t C_p \cdot dt + A(t)_t/V_p \tag{45}$$

$$A(\infty)/V_p = k_{10} \int_0^\infty C_p \cdot dt \tag{46}$$

from the equations (45) and (46)

$$A(t)/A(\infty) = (C_p + k_{10} \int_0^t C_p \cdot dt + A(t)_t/V_p)/(k_{10} \int_0^\infty C_p \cdot dt) \tag{47}$$

The terms $C(t)_p$, $Cp \cdot dt$ and $Cp \cdot dt$ are obtained from oral study. On the other hand, k_{10} is to be obtained from i.v. study. The term $A(t)_t/V_p$, which can be obtained by using a complex mathematical approximation procedure (not discussed here), requires both oral and i.v. data

$$A(t)_t/V_p = ((A(0)_t)/V_p) \cdot e^{-k_{21}\Delta t} + (k_{12}/k_{21}) \cdot C(0)_p \cdot (1 - e^{-k_{21}\Delta t}) + k_{12} \cdot (\Delta C/\Delta t)(\Delta t)^2/2 \tag{48}$$

where

A_p = amount of drug in the plasma compartment
A_t = amount of drug in the tissue compartment
$A(t)_p$ = amount of drug in plasma compartment at time t
$A(t)_t$ = amount of drug in tissue compartment at time t
$A(0)_t$ = amount of drug in tissue compartment at time 0
$C(t)_p$ = plasma drug concentration at time t and
$C(0)_p$ = plasma drug concentration at time 0

Model problem 7

The following are the plasma concentrations of a drug whose kinetics are best described by two compartment open model, in a normal healthy subject after 20 mg p.o. Estimate the absorption rate constant (k_a) using Loo-Riegelman method. The values of k_{12}, k_{21}, k_{10} and λ_z (terminal elimination rate) calculated from the i.v. data in the same subject are 0.017, 0.024, 0.015 and 0.0077 min^{-1} respectively.

```
*************************************************
***  Absorption rate  by Loo-Riegelman method  ***
*************************************************
```

term1	term2	term3	term4	term5
0	0	0	.31875	.31875
.31875	.2827059	.6007351	.22525	1.108691
1.108691	.8721274	1.934574	.5440001	3.350702
3.350702	2.635755	2.901861	.238	5.775616
5.775616	4.543261	3.325049	6.799995E-02	7.93631
7.93631	4.910857	6.156648	-.17	10.89751
10.89751	2.581922	11.78311	-3.519	10.84603
10.84603	2.569726	8.053592	-2.754	7.869318
7.869318	1.86446	5.134841	-1.785	5.2143
5.2143	1.235413	3.243057	-1.122	3.35647
3.35647	.7952409	2.053936	-.714	2.135177

Area under the curve (0-inf) = 4195.189 ug/ml/min

Given data (from i.v.study)
```
***************************
```

k12= .017 1/min
k21= .024 1/min
k10= .015 1/min

time	conc	term6	k10*auc	At/Ainf	% unabsorbed
5	7.5	8.100001	.28125	.1287189	87.12811
10	12.8	14.95119	1.0425	.2375927	76.24073
20	19.2	25.9932	3.4425	.4130637	58.69363
30	22	34.30812	6.5325	.5451979	45.48022
40	22.8	40.62881	9.8925	.6456414	35.43586
60	21.8	49.28001	16.5825	.7831195	21.68806
120	14.9	58.84353	33.0975	.9350956	6.490445
180	9.5	61.44682	44.0775	.9764649	2.353507
240	6	62.2668	51.0525	.9894955	1.050448
300	3.8	62.61897	55.4625	.9950918	.4908204
360	2.4	62.78768	58.2525	.9977728	.2227187

No.	Time (min)	Log(% unabs)	Exp(Y)	(Exp-Obs)^2
1	5	4.46738	4.196466	7.339444E-02
2	10	4.333896	4.111489	.0494646
3	20	4.072331	3.941537	1.710721E-02
4	30	3.817277	3.771584	2.087908E-03
5	40	3.567724	3.601631	1.149664E-03
6	60	3.076762	3.261725	3.421148E-02
7	120	1.870331	2.242008	.1381438
8	180	.8559066	1.222291	.1342377
9	240	4.921716E-02	.2025743	.0235184
10	300	-.711677	-.8171425	1.112297E-02
11	360	-1.501846	-1.83686	.1122344

slope of regression line=-1.699528E-02
sum of sqr.deviations= .5966726
correlation coeff.=-.9936551
Absorption rate ka = 1.699528E-02

Time (min)	Conc (μg/mL)	Time (min)	Conc (μg/mL)
5	7.5	60	21.8
10	12.8	120	14.9
20	10.2	180	9.5
30	22.0	240	6.0
40	22.8	300	3.8
		360	2.4

Solution:

term $1 = A(0)_t)/V_p$
term $2 = (A(0)_t/V_p) \cdot e^{-k_{21}\Delta t}$
term $3 = (k_{12}/k_{21}) \cdot C(0)_p \cdot (1 - e^{-k_{21}\Delta t})$
term $4 = k_{12} \cdot (\Delta C/\Delta t)\,(\Delta t)^2/2$
term $5 = A(t)_t/V_p$
term $6 = k_{10} \int_0^t C_p \cdot dt.$

3 Distribution

Following absorption, drug which enters blood circulation is distributed in the entire body. Free as well as protein bound forms undergo distribution. Distribution into specific tissues occurs depending on the physico-chemical properties of the drug and the affinity between the drug molecule and different cell structures (e.g. deposition of tetracyclines in teeth, antineoplastic substances on DNA and clofazimine in sub-cutaneous fat). The extent of vasculature and blood supply also play an important role and they may even decide the rate of distribution. Some anatomically peculiar cell membranes act as barriers and may often selectively hinder permeability of drugs. For example, the blood brain barrier (BBB) hinders transportation of water soluble drugs into brain. Similarly high molecular weight substances such as heparin and plasma expanders are prevented to cross the placental barrier, whereas other substances are allowed. Only the unbound form of drug can penetrate the cells and the bound form is prevented entry by cell limiting structures. This explains why only the free form is excreted in saliva and sweat and why protein binding restricts the distribution of drugs so much.

The most important aspect that controls drug action is the availability of active substance in sufficiently high concentrations at the site of action. Penetration of drug into the affected tissue or structure (e.g. cerebrospinal fluid in meningitis) is therefore essential to achieve effective drug concentrations.

3.1 Plasma protein binding

Drug in blood circulation may exist in two forms, bound and unbound (free). The extent of protein binding can be as low as 1% (e.g. caffeine) or as high as 99% (e.g. warfarin). Albumin is an important binding protein which has an affinity especially for neutral as well as acidic drugs. It is synthesized in liver and distributed both intra- and extra-vascularly. It is eliminated with a half-life of 17–18 days. Basic drugs are also bound to an protein called acidic α-1-glycoprotein (AAG). In addition, some drugs are known to be bound to lipoproteins.

Equilibrium between the bound and free drug is usually established within a very short time. The interaction between the drug and the protein (albumin) is reversible and can be expressed in the form of the following equation

$$\mathrm{Alb} + \mathrm{D} \underset{k_2}{\overset{k_1}{\rightleftharpoons}} \mathrm{Alb} - \mathrm{D} \qquad (49)$$

$$(\mathrm{Alb} - \mathrm{D})/(\mathrm{Alb}) \cdot (\mathrm{D}) = (k_1/k_2) = K_A \qquad (49\,a)$$

or

$$(k_2/k_1)=K_D$$

where K_A and K_D are association and dissociation constants respectively.

K_A characterizes the affinity between drug and albumin. The above reaction is dependent on both reacting substances. Albumin in blood helps not only in transporting the drug but also in serving as a depot. As the free or unbound fraction is removed from circulation by elimination and/or distribution into tissues, more drug is dissociated from this albumin-drug complex (depot). Since albumin itself is a large molecule (MW: 68,000 D) the albumin-drug complex cannot cross the plasma membrane. As a result of this, distribution and elimination (glomerular filtration and biotransformation) of drugs which are strongly protein bound are greatly restricted. The binding sites on proteins are occupied not only by drug molecules but also by different endogenous ligands such as hormones, bilirubin, free fatty acids etc. These substances may compete with drug molecules for the same binding sites and cause interactions.

Plasma protein binding of drugs is altered in various disease states (see page 31) due to qualitative and quantitative changes in binding sites of the protein.

The (patho)-physiological changes in plasma protein binding can have clinical relevance, provided that the following criteria are fulfilled.

(a) The drug in question must have a narrow therapeutic range.
(b) There must be a direct relationship between drug concentration (unbound) and its activity.
(c) The apparent volume of distribution (see page 33) must be less than 2 L/kg.
(d) The plasma protein binding of drug must be more than 80% (free fraction $f_u < 0.2$; see Table 1).
(e) The binding sites are saturable in therapeutic concentrations.
(f) The elimination is of restricted type i.e.; depends on the free fraction (see page 49).

From Table 1, it can be seen that the drugs amitriptyline, desimipramine, digitoxin, disopyramide, imipramine, nortriptyline, phenytoin, phenylbutazone, salicylic acid, tolbutamide, valproic acid and warfarin might pose problems. The free plasma concentrations can be calculated from f_u and the total measured plasma concentration C using the relationship

$$C_u = C \cdot f_u . \tag{50}$$

3.1.1 *(Patho)-physiological changes in protein binding*

Table 2 shows different disease states during which a reduction in the albumin concentration is observed. Similarly the levels of α_1-acid glycoprotein (AAG) are influenced (increased or decreased) depending on (patho)-physiological conditions.

Table 1. Plasma protein binding of different drugs

Drug	Group	% bound	Protein
Amitriptyline	B	95	A, AAG, LP
Bupivacaine	B	90	A, AAG
Carbamazepine	N	80	A, (AAG?)
Chlordiazepoxide	B	97	A
Chlorpromazine	B	89	A, AAG, LP
Clonazepam	B	82	A
Desipramine	B	90	A, AAG, LP
Diazepam	B	98	A
Digitoxin	N	93	A
Disopyramide	B	66–81 *	A, AAG
Imipramine	B	92	A, AAG, LP
Lidocaine	B	70	A, AAG
Nortriptyline	B	92	A, AAG
Phenytoin	Ac	92	A
Phenylbutazone	Ac	97–99 *	A
Propranolol	B	92	A, AAG, LP
Quinidine	B	85	A, AAG, LP
Salicylic acid	Ac	80–95 *	A
Tolbutamide	Ac	93	A
Valproic acid	Ac	75–95 *	A
Verapamil	B	90	A, AAG, LP
Warfarin	Ac	99	A

* Concentration dependent binding.
B, base; *Ac*, acid; *N*, neutral; *A*, albumin; *AAG*, acidic α_1-glycoprotein; *LP*, lipoproteins.

Table 2. Patho-physiological changes in plasma protein binding

Albumin ↓	AAG ↑	AAG ↓
Burns	Burns	Oral contraceptives
Renal insufficiency	Kidney transplantation	Pregnancy
Liver diseases	Infections	Newborns
Inflammations	Chronic inflammatory bowel diseases	
Nephrotic syndrome	Injuries	
Cardiac insufficiency	Myocardial infarction	
Post operative phase	Post operative phase	
Undernourishment	Chronic pain	
Cancer	Cancer	
Newborns		
Pregnancy		
Geriatric patients		

The percentages of protein binding, given in Table 2 are the mean values from different studies. Age dependent changes as for example a fall in albumin concentration with a simultaneous rise in AAG in old age, must be differentiated from pathological influences. Similarly the binding of certain drugs such as thiopental, etomidate and phenytoin is reduced in geriatric patients.

In newborns, the binding of diazepam and phenytoin has been found to be lower. Interestingly albumin in infants appears to be qualitatively different from that in adults. The binding of lidocaine, bupivacaine and propranolol is comparatively low in fetus because of lower levels of AAG. Under different conditions of tissue damage (e.g. acute myocardial infarction, following surgical operations, severe burns) the AAG and lipoprotein concentrations are increased, which in turn may increase the binding of drugs like propranolol, lidocaine, disopyramide, imipramine and quinidine.

Three different specific binding sites on human serum albumin have been characterized for diazepam, digitoxin and warfarin.

In renal failure, a reduction in protein binding of all acidic drugs is observed (e.g. phenytoin, valproic acid, phenylbutazone, salicyclic acid, warfarin). Similarly the binding of numerous basic drugs (e.g. propranolol, quinidine, verapamil, diazepam, oxazepam) is also more or less reduced. There are various reasons for this reduction which include

(a) reduced serum albumin concentration,
(b) structural and functional alterations in albumin,
(c) displacement by accumulated endogenous substances at the binding sites and
(d) loss of albumin through albuminuria (particularly in nephrotic syndrome).

In liver diseases such as hepatitis or cirrhosis the protein binding is affected because of loss of albumin. In addition, restricted synthesis of albumin and increased levels of bilirubin are also responsible for reduction in protein binding of numerous substances (e.g. phenytoin, quinidine, propranolol, verapamil, many benzodiazepines).

3.2 Tissue binding

The binding of drugs in tissues which contain large amounts of protein, is of considerable importance. About 54–64% of total albumin is in extravascular compartments. Skin and muscle tissues contain fairly large amounts of albumin, 18 and 15% respectively. Because of relatively poor accessibility of tissues for investigations, not much information is available about the tissue binding of drugs. A drug binding protein (γ-protein) with a molecular weight of 42,000 D was identified in hepatic cellular fluid (about 4%) which has also been subsequently found in the tubular cells of kidneys and intestinal mucosa. There are drugs which are bound to the DNA of cell nucleus (e.g. antineoplastic drugs). Other specific binding sites include teeth and bones (e.g. tetracyclines),

Na/K-ATPase (e.g. digitalis glycosides) and dihydrofolate reductase (e.g. methotrexate).

Estimates of the extent of tissue binding can be indirectly provided by computing the volume of distribution.

3.3 Distribution volume

The expression "distribution volume or volume of distribution (V)" was first introduced in 1934 by Dominguez. This term does not refer to a real distribution volume of drug which is restricted to the total body water. It is merely a volume term or constant used to relate the plasma concentration to the amount of drug in the body, hence it is more appropriate to use the term "apparent volume of distribution".

Apparent volume of distribution gives an idea about the extent of distribution of drug into various compartments of the body. It can be as small as 5 L for a drug which is exclusively confined to the circulatory system and can be larger (10–40 L) for a drug which is widely distributed in the body. For some drugs it can exceed even the body weight (100 L or more). This indicates that the drug is bound to certain tissues or stored somewhere in the body (e.g. fat). In a situation where the drug is uniformly distributed in the body and the elimination is taking place according to linear kinetics, the concentration C is proportional to the amount of drug in the body

$$C \sim D$$

$$C = D/V \quad \text{and} \quad V = D/C(0) \tag{51}$$

The above equation, however, is applicable only to drugs which are rapidly and uniformly distributed following i.v. administration and thus follow single compartment model kinetics. The initial concentration C(0) is the ratio between the administered dose D and the volume of distribution V.

Model problem 8

Using the data of model problem 1 (see page 6), estimate

(1) apparent volume of distribution (V) and

(2) V per kg body weight.

Solution:

(1) $V = D/C(0) = 500{,}000/42 = 11{,}905$ mL

(2) 0.17 L/kg

For many drugs the assumption of single compartment model may be insufficient when it is actually required to describe the kinetics according to two compartment model (see page 7). The material transport between the distribution compartments (central and peripheral) takes place as described by the rate constants k_{12} and k_{21}. Now the volume of distribution is characterized not by one but two terms namely V_p or V_c and V_t corresponding to plasma (central) and tissue compartments respectively.

There are different methods of estimation of the volume of distribution. All computations should be based on data obtained following i.v. administration as it is seldom possible to know the exact portion of the dose that has been absorbed or reached circulation following extravascular administration.

The estimation of V by the method of extrapolation using C(0) (Y-axis intercept of concentration-time curve) is valid only for drugs whose kinetics are best described by one compartment model. Application of this method to drugs whose kinetics are described by multi-compartment model may result in over-estimation because the assumed value of C(0) in such an instance is lower than the actual one.

(1) V_{extr}: Volume of distribution, calculated ignoring the distribution phase (as in single compartment model) is known as V_{extr} which is given by the expression

$$V_{extr} = D(\text{i.v.})/C_z \tag{52}$$

V_{extr} is always the largest among different volume terms.

(2) V_{ss}: In case of a two compartment open model at the time of steady state condition, when no mass transfer takes place between the two compartments and the system is in a state of equilibrium, the volume term called "steady state volume of distribution (V_{ss})" can be calculated using Riegelman's equation

$$V_{ss} = V_p \cdot ((k_{12} + k_{21})/k_{21}) \tag{53}$$

where

$$V_p = D/C(0) = D/(C_1 + C_z) \tag{54}$$

at time $t = 0$,

$$C(0) = C_1 + C_z \tag{55}$$

V_{ss} is meaningful only at the time when the system is in a steady state and it is not so often used as a proportionality factor (concentration-mass ratio). However, it has an advantage that it is the volume term which is independent of elimination process. One should always compute V_{ss} whenever the volume of distribution has to be compared among different patient groups in a study, because in such studies one does not know whether the patients under study show differences in elimination of the drug and whether the difference in volume of distribution (which actually depends upon the elimination differences) is caused by changes in elimination.

(3) V_z: The volume term V_z is defined as a proportionality factor that corresponds to the situation after the so called "pseudo distribution equilibrium" i.e., during the terminal λ_z-phase. V is a function of time until this equilibrium is attained and at time $t = 0$, V is identical to V_p

$$V_z = V_p \cdot k_{10}/\lambda_z \tag{56}$$

In case of a two compartment open model the term clearance is defined as a product of V_p and k_{10}. The above equation can now be written as

$$V_z = CL/\lambda_z \tag{57}$$

On the other hand, clearance (CL) as a model independent parameter can be calculated using the following equation

$$CL = D(i.v.)/AUC \tag{58}$$

from the equations (57) and (58)

$$V_z = D(i.v.)/\lambda_z \cdot AUC \tag{59}$$

Gibaldi showed that the volume of distribution calculated using the equations (56), (57) or (59) is identical. In the literature, this term is frequently quoted as Vd_β or Vd_{area} and the expression V_z is according to the new nomenclature. If it is required to know the total amount of drug present in the body at any given time, V_z is the expression of choice.

The calculated volume terms will always be in the following order of magnitude

$$V_{extr} > V_z > V_{ss} > V_p$$

Model problem 9

Using the data of model problem 3 (see page 13), estimate

(1) steady state volume of distribution (V_{ss}),
(2) volume of distribution (V_z),
(3) volume of central compartment (V_p) and
(4) vomume of distribution (V_{extr}).

Solution:

(1) $V_{ss} = V_p \cdot k_{10}/\lambda_z = 25.5 \times 0.53/0.126 = 107.3$ L
(2) $V_z = D(i.v.)/\lambda_z \cdot AUC = 20{,}000{,}000/(0.126 \times 1352.5) = 117.4$ L
(3) $V_p = D/C_1 + C_z = 20{,}000{,}000/(630 + 155) = 25.5$ L
(4) $V_{extr} = D(i.v.)/C_z = 20{,}000{,}000/155 = 129$ L.

For drugs which are not appreciably bound to tissues or proteins, the apparent volume is nearly the same as the true volume of distribution. As many drugs are bound (intra- or extra-vascular), the apparent volume differs significantly from the true volume. Drugs which are strongly bound to plasma proteins have smaller apparent volume and on the other hand, drugs which are bound to extravascular tissues have larger volumes than real volumes of distribution (Table 3). Drugs with greater lipid solubility exhibit better penetration into tissues where they are bound to the proteins, hence a larger volume of distribution. This condition results in higher concentrations of drug in tissues than in plasma. Since only unbound drug is biologically active and capable of distribution into various compartments, it is more meaningful to calculate the V of free fraction.

Table 3. Fluid space in human body

Compartment	Body weight [%]	Total body water [%]
Plasma	4.5	7.5
Total extracellular water	27.0	45.0
Total intracellular water	33.0	55.0
Total body water	60.0	100.0

As mentioned before, the lower the plasma protein binding the greater is the apparent volume of distribution of free fraction (f_u) as relatively large portion of the drug can be distributed into peripheral compartment. An equilibrium is rapidly established between the free drug concentrations in plasma and tissues. The equation for the concentration of unbound fraction (f_u) is

$$C_u = C_p \cdot f_{pu} = C_t \cdot f_{tu} \tag{60}$$

where C_p and C_t are concentrations in plasma and tissue respectively.

Gillette's equation for apparent volume of distribution is

$$V_{ss} = V_p + V_t \cdot (f_{pu}/f_{tu}) \tag{61}$$

where V_p is the plasma volume (approximately 2.5 L/75 kg)

V_t is "tissue volume" (40 L/75 kg)

f_{pu} and f_{tu} are free fractions of drug in plasma and tissue compartments respectively.

There is another approach (method of statistical moments) for the calculation of apparent volume of distribution which is independent of the pharmacokinetic model. According to this method

$$V_{ss} = D(\text{i.v.}) \cdot \text{AUMC}/(\text{AUC})^2 \tag{62}$$

where AUMC is the area under the first statistical moment curve, which is the product of time t and plasma concentration C from time $t = 0$ to ∞

$$\text{AUMC} = \int_0^\infty t \cdot C\,dt \tag{63}$$

As in the case of other calculation methods, the time of sampling, analytical precision and identification of the beginning of terminal log-linear phase play important roles.

3.3.1 Factors influencing volume of distribution

Depending on the administered dose and the rate of elimination plasma concentrations are inversely proportional to the volume of distribution. It is often possible that the concentrations may be unexpectedly high, reaching toxic levels in patients with reduced volume of distribution due to some patho-physiological reasons. We have already seen that the protein binding plays a very significant role in affecting the volume of distribution and diseases of liver and kidney can influence V by altering protein binding (see page 31).

Body weight has a direct influence on V. It is often observed that V of different subjects of the same age group shows a considerable variation due to difference in body weight. It is hence customary to express V per kg of body weight to eliminate such variation. For many drugs no exact relationship exists between these two factors, because the gain in body weight is often due to increase in body fat or water instead of muscle (protein). This change in the overall composition of the body can potentially influence the nature of distribution.

In adults (age range: 18–55 years), the body fat content increases with age from 18 to 36% for men and 33 to 48% for women respectively. On the other hand, the total body water in newborn is 70 to 75% of the body weight and it reaches the adult value of 60% at the age of 13 years. Similarly the extracellular water content in newborn is about 40%, which gradually reduces to about 25% at the age of 13 years. Thus it is evident that age and sex have a considerable influence on V of drugs and there are several interesting examples in the literature which elicit the influence of age on drug action. Volume of distribution of diazepam for example increases with age and that of antipyrine, pethidine and propacillin decreases. A significant increase in V of digoxin in newborn and infants upto 7 months can be noticed.

Physical stress through heat and motion can also affect V as it alters blood perfusion to different organs and body hydration.

Blood flow and cardiac output also play a major role in affecting the distribution of drugs. The distribution of volatile anaesthetics like halothane and isoflurane is dependent on the cardiac output (which goes down by about 1% every year from 19 to 86 years). Similarly in congestive heart failure V is altered because of changes in perfusion (e.g. procainamide, lidocaine).

V can also be changed due to drug interactions. For example, probenecid affects the pharmacokinetics of penicillin by reducing its excretion and increasing V.

Similarly in many disease states a change in V is noticed. In renal diseases (e.g. uremia, nephrotic syndrome) reduced protein binding of phenytoin results in increased V. However, if V is calculated for unbound phenytoin no significant changes will emerge. It is assumed that in patients with renal failure, a reduction in V of drugs which are essentially excreted unchanged in urine is a general phenomenon. There are several examples for this observation which include methotrexate, cephalexin, colistimethate, lincomycin, methicillin, insulin and digoxin. In case of digoxin, besides slower elimination a reduction in volume of distribution may lead to toxic plasma levels.

In liver diseases, often a reduction in plasma protein binding which results in increased V is observed (e.g. diazepam, propranolol). Antibiotics like penicillin and gentamicin diffuse better into CNS in a pathological condition such as meningitis than in normal condition, probably because of increased permeability of blood brain barrier (BBB) due to inflammation.

4 Elimination

The duration of action and removal of drug from the body are determined by elimination processes. As soon as the drug appears in blood, its transportation to organs of elimination (e.g. liver, kidneys, lungs, intestines, skin and salivary glands) begins. Elimination includes not only the process of excretion but all mechanisms that reduce the amount of drug in body. Water solubility is one of the prerequisites for drug excretion. A substance which is sufficiently water soluble is excreted essentially unchanged by the kidneys and a substance which has a limited water solubility, will undergo biotransformation into more polar molecule(s) before it can be excreted. Biotransformation or metabolism takes place primarily in liver and to a smaller extent in kidneys, muscles and intestines. If the metabolite is still not polar enough, then part of it is reabsorbed in the renal tubules probably to undergo further metabolism. The kinetics of renal excretion can be described in the same way as hepatic elimination kinetics (1st order reaction kinetics) and the same mathematical equations can be applied (see page 4).

4.1 Half-life and clearance

Similar to radioactive decomposition fall in drug concentration in the body can be quantitatively described using the term "biological or elimination half-life ($t_{1/2}$)", which is defined as the time required for the concentration to fall to one half after the distribution equilibrium is attained. As the concentration refers to drug in plasma, the elimination half-life is also called as "plasma half-life".

As the elimination in plasma takes place according to the 1st order rate kinetics, the rate of change or fall in concentration is proportional to the concentration of the drug at time t (see page 4).

$$-dC/dt \sim C$$

(or)

$$-dC/dt = k \cdot C \tag{1}$$

integrating the above differential equation from time 0 to t

$$-\int_0^t dC/C = k \cdot \int_0^t dt$$

$$\ln C(0)/C(t) = k \cdot t$$

or

$$C(t) = C(0) \cdot e^{-k \cdot t} \tag{2}$$

according to definition

$$t_{1/2} = 0.693/k. \tag{3}$$

This reciprocal relationship between k and $t_{1/2}$ is valid only in case of one compartment model (see page 6). In case of two compartment model, during the more rapid disposition (distribution) phase

$$t_{1/2\,\lambda_1} = 0.693/\lambda_1 \tag{3a}$$

and during the terminal (elimination) phase

$$t_{1/2\,\lambda_z} = 0.693/\lambda_z \tag{3b}$$

For accurate determination of half-life one requires sufficient number of data points on the time-concentration curve so that the terminal phase is well characterized. One can also determine $t_{1/2}$ using the following relationships

1-compartment open model:

$$t_{1/2} = 0.693 \cdot V/CL \tag{64}$$

2-compartment open model:

$$t_{1/2} = 0.693 \cdot V_z/CL. \tag{64a}$$

It is obvious from these equations that half-life can be altered by changes not only in clearance but also in volume of distribution.

Clearance is the most suitable term that characterizes elimination. It can be defined as "the volume of plasma or blood cleared from drug in unit time". Clearance of a drug, as mentioned previously takes place through different routes including mainly kidneys (renal clearance CL_R) and liver (hepatic clearance CL_H). Clearance which is measurable from plasma data represents total body clearance (sum of renal, hepatic, pulmonary and biliary clearances)

$$CL = CL_R + CL_H + CL_X + \dots \tag{65}$$

and (overall) elimination rate constant is the sum of individual rates.

$$k = k_e \text{ (urinary excretion rate)} + k_m \text{ (metabolic rate)} + k_x + \dots$$

Total clearance can be computed as a model independent parameter using the following equation

$$CL = D(\text{i.v.})/AUC = F \cdot D(\text{p.o.})/AUC \tag{66}$$

where $F(=f_a \cdot f_{fp})$ is the bioavailability of drug following extravascular (e.v.) administration which is a product of fraction absorbed (f_a) and the fraction of absorbed amount that has not been removed by a first-pass effect (f_{fp}) (see page 52).

Model problem 10

Using the data of model problems 1 (see page 5) and 3 (see page 13) estimate total body clearance (CL) of the new drug and famotidine respectively.

Solution:

(1) $CL = k \cdot V = 0.25 \times 11.9 = 2.98$ L/h

(or) $CL = D/AUC = 500{,}000/179.98 = 2.78$ L/h

(2) $CL = k_{10} \cdot V_p = 0.53 \times 25.5 = 13.5$ L/h

(or) $CL = 0.693 \times V_z/t_{1/2} = 0.693 \times 117.4/5.5 = 14.8$ L/h

In majority of cases depending on the chemical nature of drug, elimination occurs exclusively either through renal route or through hepatic route. The elimination is said to be predominant hepatic type when less than about 250% of the administered dose is excreted unchanged in urine and the rest is eliminated by liver. On the other hand, it is known as predominant renal type if most part of the administered dose is excreted unchanged in urine. The total body clearance CL calculated from plasma data represents CL_H in the first instance and CL_R in the latter. However, it is required to compute the individual clearances separately in a situation where both liver and kidneys contribute to the total clearance. From the cumulative urinary excretion data one can determine CL_R, provided that the amount excreted upto 4 to 5 half-lives (A_e^∞) and AUC are known

$$A_e^\infty/D = k_e/k \quad \text{or} \quad k_e = A_e^\infty \cdot k/D \tag{67}$$

$$CL_R = A_e^\infty/AUC = A_e^\infty \cdot CL/D \tag{68}$$

and

$$CL_H = CL - CL_R \tag{68 a}$$

The equations for calculating clearance in different kinetic models are given below

1-compartment open model:

$$CL = k \cdot V \text{ (from equation 64)} \tag{69}$$

2-compartment open model:

$$CL = k \cdot V_p = k_{10} \cdot V_p \tag{70}$$

$$CL = \lambda_z \cdot V_z = 0.693 \cdot V_z/t_{1/2} \tag{71}$$

(from equation 64 a)

In equation (70) it is assumed that elimination ($k_{10} = k$) takes place from central compartment (V_p)

4.2 Renal elimination

Drugs which are sufficiently water soluble are excreted unchanged in urine. They are essentially excreted by glomerular filtration similar to endogenous creatinine. Drugs with residual lipid solubility are reabsorbed in the renal tubules (e.g. barbiturates). In addition to glomerular filtration active tubular secretion with the help of carriers also takes place in kidneys (e.g. penicillin,

H_2-receptor antagonists). Two different carrier systems, one for acidic and the other for basic drugs have been characterized. The amount of drug which is ultimately excreted in urine depends upon all these three mechanisms.

+glomerular filtration
+tubular secretion
−tubular reabsorption

=net amount excreted

Tubular reabsorption is influenced by pH of urine and body posture. It also shows circadian fluctuations. The reabsorption and active secretion can be controlled by altering the pH of urine (e.g. alkalisation by coadministration of bicarbonate). By increasing the degree of ionisation (improved water solubility) the extent of reabsorption can be minimized.

Dissociation of acidic drugs (e.g. salicylates) having a pKa value between 3 and 6 is strongly influenced by pH fluctuations in urine. Substances with a pKa value less than 2 essentially remain ionised at any pH of urine. Reabsorption of basic drugs (e.g. amphetamine) with a pKa value between 7.5 and 10.5 is greatly affected by changes in pH of urine.

In case of barbiturate poisoning alkalisation of urine enhances the excretion of the ionised form through reduced reabsorption. Similarly acidification can as well enhance the excretion of basic drugs like pethidine and morphine (more examples are given in Table 4).

The elimination through kidneys depends essentially upon the renal blood flow. Kidney function is best characterized by creatinine clearance and the latter can be calculated by taking the amount of creatinine excreted in 24 h and serum creatinine concentration at the mid-point of time of urine collection into account. In practice it is also possible and more simple to employ the estimated serum creatinine value. A non-linear correlation exists between both values.

There are different nomograms (see for example Fig. 6) and formulae for the calculation of creatinine clearance. Besides, it is important to notice that age, body weight and sex have a significant influence on creatinine clearance. Equations (72) to (74) are the formulae for calculation of creatinine clearance (CL_{cr} in man.

for men

$$CL_{cr}(\text{mL/min}) = (140 - \text{age}) \cdot \text{wt}/72 \cdot \text{serum creatinine (mg/100 mL)} \quad (72)$$

for women

$$CL_{cr}(\text{mL/min}) = 0.85 \cdot (CL_{cr})_{men} \quad (73)$$

(or)

$$CL_{cr}(\text{mL/min}) = (140 - \text{age}) \cdot \text{wt}/85 \cdot \text{serum creatinine (mg/100 mL)} \quad (73\,a)$$

for children

$$CL_{cr} = 0.55 \cdot \text{height/serum creatinine} \quad (74)$$

Table 4. Drugs, whose tubular reabsorption is affected by reverse diffusion in unionised form and excretion of which can be altered in urine through alkalization or acidification (Anderson 1981, Gladtke 1973)

Weak acids	Weak bases
Acetazolamide	Adrenalin
Aminoacids	Amphetamine
p-Aminobenzoic acid	Chloroquine
Barbital	
Bromocresol green	Codeine
Bromophenol blue	Dexamphetamine
Carbutamide	Dopamine
Cephaloridine	
Citric acid	Flecainide
Dinitrophenol	
Ethacrynic acid	5-Hydroxytryptamine
Furosemide	Levorphanol
Hydrochlorthiazide	Meperidine
Indole acetic acid	Morphine
Mersalyl	Neostigmine
Methotrexate	Nicotine
Nitrofurantoin	Pethidine
p-Aminohippuric acid	Procaine
Penicillin	Quinacrine
Phenobarbital	Quinidine
Phenol red	Quinine
Phenylbutazone	Santoquine
Probenicid	Thiamine
Salicylic acid	Tricyclic antidepressants
Sulfonamides	Trimethoprim

Model problem 11

What is the creatinine clearance in a man (57 years) weighing 75 kg, if his serum creatinine concentration is 0.85 mg/dL?

Solution:

$$\begin{aligned} CL_{cr}(\text{mL/min}) &= (140-\text{age}) \cdot \text{wt}/72 \cdot \text{serum creatinine (mg/100 mL)} \\ &= (140-57) \times 75/72 \times 0.85 \\ &= 6225/61.2 = 101.7 \text{ mL/min.} \end{aligned}$$

In newborn and infants (up to 2 months) the renal elimination does not reach its full capacity because the glomerular filtration rate, GFR (characterized by inulin clearance) is only about 10 mL/min (the adult value is 120 mL/min from 5 months). Filtration and tubular secretion together (determined through p-aminohippuric acid clearance) amount to only 25 mL/min (the adult value is 650 mL/min from 7 months). Thus it may be expected that the elimination of drugs can show a marked variation in the age group of 1 to 6 months. The clearance of digoxin for example in 1-month old babies is 53 mL/min/1.73 m^2 and in 4–6 month old babies 87 mL/min/1.73 m^2.

In reduced renal function with apparently high serum creatinine levels (over 1.5 mg/100 mL), the drug clearance in general is reduced ($t_{1/2}$ is prolonged). In an extreme situation like anuria, only extrarenal elimination takes place and excretion in feces may be relatively increased to compensate the impaired renal clearance.

The relationship between renal function and elimination can be best explained by Dettli's equation

$$k = k_m + \alpha' \cdot GFR \tag{75}$$

and for the half-life

$$t_{1/2} = 0.693/(k_m + \alpha' \cdot GFR) \tag{76}$$

where the proportionality factor α' relates renal drug elimination to GFR; k_m can be considered as zero when the drug is excreted unchanged. On the other hand, in anuria for a drug which is partly eliminated through liver $k = k_m$. In this condition some drugs (e.g. doxycycline, gentamicin) are excreted extrarenally. In case of aminoglycosides, however, the half-life is very much prolonged (see Table 5) due to exclusion of renal elimination.

In Table 5 the half-lives of different drugs in renal failure (right column) are given. Reduced elimination due to restricted renal function leads to accumulation of drug in the body following multiple or repeated administration and the associated risk of toxic effects is also increased. This problem can be prevented by adjusting or suitably altering the dosage regimen of the drug depending on the extent of renal failure. There are three possible methods of doing this:

(1) by increasing the dosing interval without altering the normal dose.

(2) for certain drugs (e.g. penicillins, cephalosporins, aminoglycosides) it is often recommended to reduce the maintenance dose to half the initial dose and the dosing interval is estimated from formula (Kunin's rule)

$$\tau = t_{1/2}/Q^* \tag{77}$$

where Q^* is the correction factor.

(3) reducing the maintenance dose without altering the dosing interval.

The latter is in general preferable because the fluctuations in plasma concentration-time profile are smaller during a dosing interval.

The correction factor Q^*, with which the normal dose must be multiplied or τ must be divided, can be obtained with the help of the scheme given in Fig. 6. However, the extent of extrarenal elimination must be known. This value is expressed as percentage by multiplying the ratio $k_m/k = Q_0$ by 100 (see Table 5).

A drug which is predominantly (say 90%) excreted unchanged in urine, has a Q_0 value of 0.1 which implies that 10% must be eliminated by extrarenal route. Between this point on the ordinate and the right-top corner a straight line is drawn. From the known serum creatinine concentration (upper abscissa) or creatinine clearance (lower abscissa) a vertical line has to be drawn which

Table 5. Elimination rate constants (and half lives) of different drugs in patients with normal renal function (k) and severely impaired renal function (k_m)

Medicament	k (h^{-1}) (normal)	k_m (h^{-1}) (in anuria)	$Q_0 = \frac{k_m}{k}$	$t_{1/2}$ (h)	
				Normal	Renal insufficiency
Ampicillin	0.8	0.05	0.12	0.9	10–18
Carbenicilline	0.6	0.06	0.1	1–1.5	12–16
Cephazoline	0.35	0.02	0.06	2.0	30
Cephalexine	0.7	0.03	0.04	1.0	14–18
Cephaloridine	0.4	0.03	0.08	1.5	20
Cephalothine	1.4	0.06	0.04	0.7	12
Chloramphenicol	0.3	0.25	0.83	2–3	3–4
Chlorpropamide	0.02	0.008	0.40	34	80–200
Chlortetracyclin	0.1	0.09	0.9	6	7–11
Clindamycin	0.25	0.2	0.8	2.5	3–5
Cloxacillin	1.2	0.31	0.26	0.6	2
Colistimethat	0.15	0.054	0.35	4.5	10–12
Dicloxacillin	1.2	0.6	0.50	0.75	1.5
Digitoxin	0.0047	0.0042	0.88	150	Unchanged
Digoxin	0.02	0.007	0.33	35–40	90–110
Doxycyclin	0.033	0.03	0.9	15–18	18–23
Erythromycin	0.5	0.13	0.26	1.4	5–6
Gentamycin	0.3	0.01	0.03	2.0	35–67
Isoniazid	0.5	0.40	0.8	1.3	
	0.25	0.13	0.5	3.0	
Kanamycin	0.3	0.01	0.03	2.5	65–96
Lidocain	0.39	0.36	0.92	1.8	Unchanged
Lincomycin	0.15	0.06	0.40	5	10–13
Methicillin	1.4	0.18	0.13	0.5	4
Methyldigoxin	0.017	0.009	0.5	43	80–100
Minocyclin	0.041	0.036	0.9	17–21	20–26
Nafcillin	1.25	0.54	0.43	0.6	1.5
Oxacillin	1.5	0.5	0.33	0.5	1
Oxytetracyclin	0.075	0.014	0.19	9.2	45–66
Penicillin G	1.4	0.07	0.05	0.5	7–10
Propranolol	0.22	0.16	0.73	3–4	Unchanged
Rifampicin	0.25	0.25	1	3	Unchanged
Streptomycin	0.25	0.01	0.04	2.5	52–100
Sulfamethoxazol	0.075	0.06	0.8	8–10	10–12
Tetracycline	0.08	0.01	0.13	8.5	57–108
Trimethoprim	0.06	0.03	0.5	9–11	20–30
Vancomycin	0.12	0.004	0.03	4–6	100–200

intercepts the diagonal straight line. From the point of interception a horizontal line is drawn to the Y-axis to obtain the desired Q* factor. This value represents relative individual elimination rate. The method is applicable only for drugs whose kinetics are described by one compartment open model and in case where the disturbances in renal function have no influence on volume of distribution and metabolism.

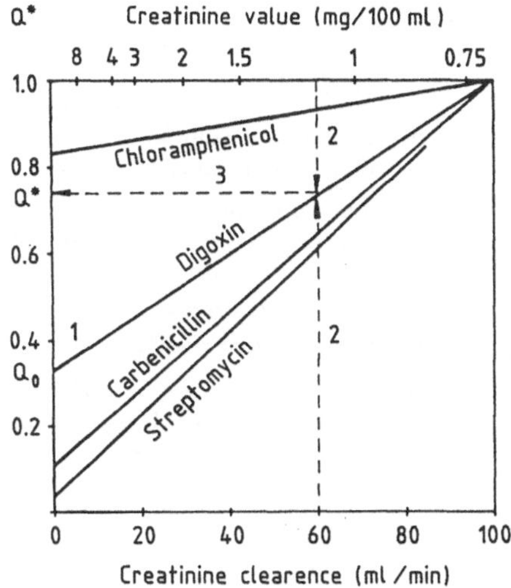

Fig. 6. Nomogram for the determination of the correction factor Q*, which enables calculation of individual maintenance dose (or dosing interval) of a drug which is eliminated through kidneys

In patients with severe renal failure often blood purification is undertaken by dialysis or hemofiltration. Under such conditions the elimination is dependent on factors as blood and dialysate or filtrate flow rate, membrane permeability or pore size and surface area of membrane. In addition, molecular size, polarity, protein binding and volume of distribution of drug play an important role. In this context the term "dialysance" (often called as extracorporeal clearance) is used to represent clearance. It is given by the equation:

$$CL_D = Q_D(C_A - C_V)/C_A \tag{78}$$

where Q_D = blood flow through the artificial kidney (dialysis machine)

C_A = arterial (into dialysis machine) concentration of drug

C_V = venous (from dialysis machine) concentration of drug.

The extracorporeal clearance can also be calculated from the expression:

$$CL_D = A_D/AUC \tag{79}$$

where A_D = amount excreted during the dialysis process, AUC = area under plasma concentration-time curve during the same period.

The total body clearance (CL_{TD}) during the period of dialysis is the sum of body clearance (CL) and dialysance (CL_D) as shown in the equation

$$CL_{TD} = CL + CL_D\,. \tag{80}$$

The fraction lost during dialysis can be calculated from the following equation

$$f_D = 1 - e^{-(CL + CL_D)\cdot(\tau/V)} \tag{81}$$

where τ is the duration of dialysis.

Table 6. Drug properties and dialysability

Properties	Dialysis characteristics
Water solubility	Water insoluble or fat soluble drugs are not dialysable (e.g. glutethimide which is practically insoluble in water).
Protein binding	Strongly bound substances are poorly dialysable as dialysis is a passive diffusion process (e.g. propranolol, which is about 94% bound).
Molecular weight	Molecules with MW < 500 D are easily dialysable (e.g. vancomycin; MW 1800 D is very poorly dialysable).
Drugs with large V	Are slowly dialysable, as most part of the drug is concentrated in the tissues (e.g. digoxin; V = 500 L is not rapidly dialysable).

In case of hemofiltration the filtration clearance (CL_{HF}) is given by the equation

$$CL_{HF} = Q_F \cdot S \tag{82}$$

where S is the sieve coefficient of the filter which may be calculated from the following formula

$$S = 2 \times C_F/(C_{in} + C_{out}) \tag{83}$$

where

C_F = concentration of drug in the filtrate
C_{in} = concentration of drug in the plasma before filtration
C_{out} = concentration of drug in the plasma after filtration.

If CL_D or CL_F is more than 30% at the end of dialysis/filtration a dosage supplementation (corresponding to the fraction eliminated) is required. Drugs with high molecular weight (e.g. vancomycin, MW = 1800; amphotericin, MW = 960) or drugs which have a very large volume of distribution (e.g. digoxin, V = 500 l) or drugs which exhibit strong protein binding (e.g. warfarin, f_u = 1%; diazepam, f_u = 2%) are poorly dialysable (also see Table 6). The amount actually removed (A_D or A_F) shows how effective the dialysis or filtration is and whether or not any dosage substitution at the end of such process is required.

Model problem 12

The plasma clearance (CL) and volume of distribution (V) of phenobarbital in a patient with renal insufficiency were 8 mL/min and 50 L respectively. Assuming a dialysis clearance of 60 mL/min how long should he be dialysed to remove 50% of drug from the body.

Solution:

$$f_D = 1 - e^{-(CL + CL_D)\cdot(\tau/V)}$$

$$0.5 = 1 - e^{-(68)(\tau/50{,}000)} \quad \text{(or)} \quad \log(0.5) = -68 \times \tau/50{,}000$$

$$\tau = 0.5\ \text{h}$$

4.3 Hepatic elimination

Metabolism or biotransformation is a process which essentially involves the conversion of a lipophilic substance into more water soluble form(s). The most important site of drug metabolism is liver and different reactions take place in subcellular structures of smooth endoplasmic reticulum ("microsomal fraction" obtained following differential centrifugation of liver cell homogenates). These reactions can be mainly divided into two categories.

(a) nonsynthetic phase I reactions: which include oxidation, hydroxylation, reduction, hydrolysis, deamination and dealkylation
(b) synthetic phase II reactions: which include (1) conjugation (coupling) of substances with glucuronic acid, sulfuric acid and glycine and (2) transfer of methyl and acetyl groups.

The phase I reactions often through creation of new functional groups (particularly hydroxyl group) enable the conjugation (phase II) reactions to take place, such that the water solubility of the first product is further increased. The product of phase I reaction is sometimes still active but after phase II or conjugation reaction, in most cases the activity is lost (one exception is morphine glucuronide). Some examples for biologically active metabolites are given in Table 7.

The mixed functional monooxidase system of phase I reactions is rather non-specific, therefore endogenous substances such as hormones, steroids and bile acids, like many drugs undergo hydroxylation. These biotransformations are of great significance. Oxidative reactions require the reduced nicotinamide-adenine-dinucleotide-phosphate (NADPH), hydrogen and cytochrome P450 (P448). This system is genetically controlled and is influenced by many factors. The postulated role of cytochrome P450 in the oxidative biotransformation is shown here.

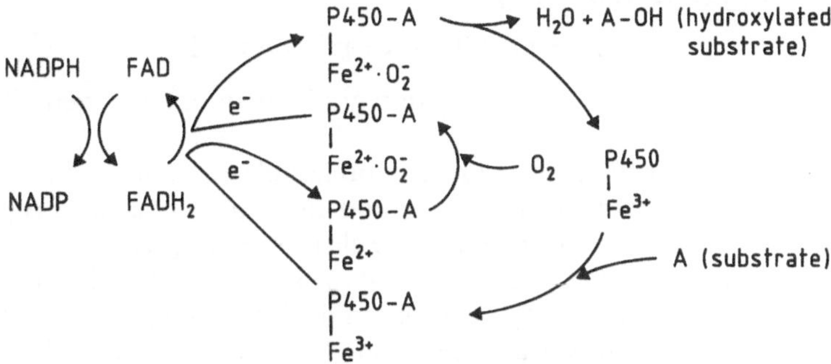

Table 7. Drugs and their biologically active metabolites (which can be used therapeutically)

Drug	Metabolite	Pharmacological effect of metabolite
Acetyldigoxin	Digoxin	Cardioactive
Allopurinol	Oxipurinol	Reduces uric acid levels
Amitryptyline	Desmethylamitryptyline	Sedative, antidepressant
Carbamazepin	Carbamazepin-10,11-epoxide	Anticonvulsant
Chloralhydrate	Trichloroethanol	Hypnotic
Codeine	Morphine	Analgesic
Diazepam	Desmethyldiazepam, Oxazepam, Temazepam	Sedative, hypnotic
Digitoxin	Digoxin	Cardioactive
Imipramine	Desmethylimipramine	Sedative, antidepressant
β-Methyldigoxin	Digoxin	Cardioactive
Phenacetin	Paracetamol	Analgesic, antipyretic
Phenylbutazone	Oxyphenylbutazone	Anti-inflammatory, antirheumatic
Primidone	Phenobarbital	Sedative, anticonvulsant

Hepatic elimination, through the influence of microsomal enzymes can be impaired when the capacity limited enzyme system is saturated with large excess of substrate. For example, administration of large doses of phenytoin results in non-linear pharmacokinetics due to reduced elimination. Drugs like sultiam, cimetidine and dicoumarol derivatives inhibit oxidative metabolism and thereby reduce the elimination of other drugs. On the other hand, many substances can enhance the elimination by stimulating or inducing protein synthesis leading to increased levels of microsomal enzymes. The most popular substances are phenobarbital, rifampicin, carbamazepin, glutethimide, steroids, DDT (insecticide) and polycyclic carbon compounds (from cigarette smoke). Accelerated metabolism (elimination) can be partly responsible for the development of tolerance to barbiturates. As a result of this induction the elimination of various endogenous substances is also hastened. The effect of an inducer reaches the peak after a pre-treatment for a few days and it gradually fades away in due course of time following discontinuation of the treatment.

Hepatic clearance can be expressed in the same way as renal clearance taking liver blood flow (Q_H) and arterial/venous blood concentration of drug across the liver into consideration (Fig. 7).

$$CL_H = Q_H \cdot (C_A - C_V)/C_A = Q_H \cdot E \tag{84}$$

where E is extraction ratio (concentration gradient across the organ of elimination).

For physiological interpretation it is preferable to express the concentrations and clearance with respect to blood instead of plasma. Liver can be considered as a dynamic system where the clearance of a given drug is essentially controlled by the rate of blood flow (Q_H) and the extraction ratio (E). A slower perfusion results in better extraction due to prolonged contact with the liver cells (partly to compensate the lowered CL_H due to reduced Q_H).

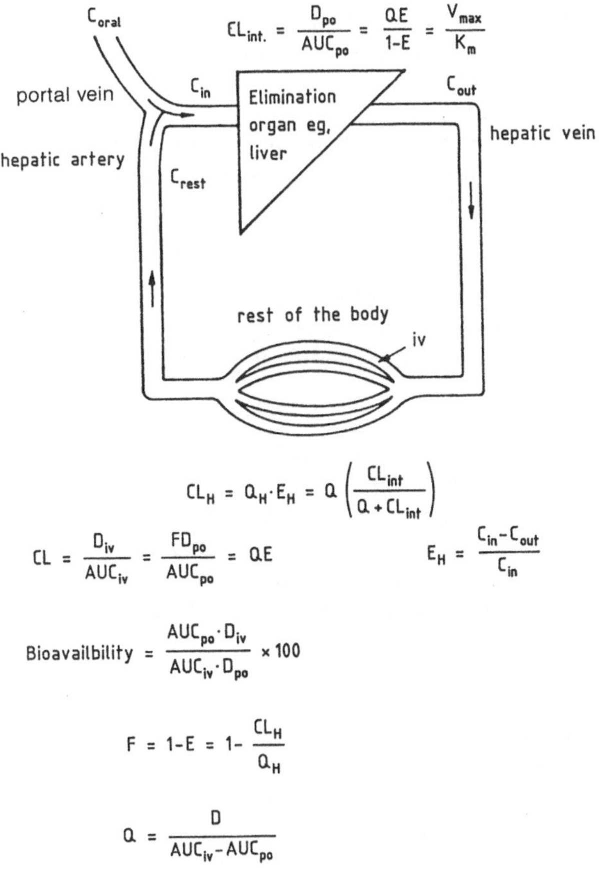

Fig. 7. The physiological clearance-concept with important pharmacokinetic formulae

Based on the hepatic blood flow (500–2500 ml/min, average: 1500 ml/min) the elimination may be divided into two types.

(1) Drugs with high hepatic clearance ($CL_H > 1000$ ml/min) show a perfusion dependent or perfusion limited elimination and the extraction ratio (E) for such drugs is greater than 0.7 (e.g. chlormethiazole, dihydroergotamine, lidocaine, metoprolol, pentazocine, propranolol and verapamil).

(2) Drugs with low hepatic clearance ($CL_H < 300$ ml) exhibit perfusion independent elimination. Here the capacity of liver enzymes (extraction ratio E is less than 0.2) plays a limited role (e.g. diazepam, digitoxin, indomethacin, theophylline, tolbutamide and valproic acid).

For numerous drugs (e.g. allopurinol, quinidine, chlorpromazine, fentanyl, ketanserine, triamterene, midazolam) the clearance is partly dependent on perfusion (intermediate to the above mentioned extreme cases).

For drugs which are strongly bound to plasma proteins (>90%), the unbound or free fraction (f_u) often affects the clearance and these drugs show restricted elimination (e.g. phenytoin, warfarin).

$$CL_H = Q_H(f_u \cdot CL_{int}/(Q_H + f_u \cdot CL_{int})) \tag{85}$$

where $CL_{int} = (Q - E)/(1 - E)$.

The intrinsic clearance represents the maximum capacity of liver, with which the drug is irreversibly removed from blood. In a situation where $CL_{int} \cdot f_u \ll Q$, the above expression is simplified to

$$CL_H = CL_{int} \cdot f_u \tag{86}$$

and the CL_H is therefore proportional to f_u.

The influence of clearance through the plasma protein binding can be eliminated when the clearance of free fraction (CL_u) is calculated using the equation

$$CL_u = CL/f_u \tag{87}$$

In contrast to this, in case of non-restrictive type of elimination the liver enzymes metabolise free as well as bound fraction of drug (e.g. propranolol, lidocaine). Most of the substances are eliminated with high CL (>800 ml/min), in which case $CL_{int} \cdot f_u \gg Q$, and CL approaches Q ($CL \sim Q$). It may be concluded that the clearance is only dependent on perfusion of the organ of elimination and the plasma protein binding is not of significance.

Since the liver perfusion represents about 25% of cardiac output, cardiac insufficiency can lead to delayed hepatic elimination of some drugs (e.g. theophylline, lidocaine).

To judge whether liver disease influences the hepatic elimination or not, one should take patient factors on one side and nature of drug on the other into consideration. Nature and severity of the disease must be clearly defined. Age, sex, smoking habit, nutritional status, comedication and accompanying diseases (e.g. cardiac insufficiency) can considerably influence drug metabolism. The extent of protein binding which is often lowered in liver diseases and pharmacokinetic behaviour of drug have to be taken into consideration for adjusting the dose in liver disease.

In hepatic dysfunction many pathophysiological changes can occur (Table 8). For example, Q_H is lowered through intra- and extra-hepatic shunts, leading to an increase in the bioavailability of high clearance drugs (see page 52). In chronic liver diseases the cell mass and function may be reduced, which simultaneously results in (reduction in E!) reduced clearance.

Table 8. Pathophysiological changes in different liver diseases

Hepatic functional disturbances	Q	Liver cell mass	Hepatocyte function
Cirrhosis			
moderate	↓	↔ ↑	↔
severe	↓↓	↓	↓
Viral hepatitis	↔ ↑	↔ ↓	↓
Alcohol hepatitis	↔ ↓	↑ ↔ ↓	↓

It was already mentioned earlier that patients with liver disease may often receive more than one drug which can possibly interact with one another. Smoking habit and nutritional status of patients should likewise be taken into consideration. Smoking has been reported to enhance hepatic elimination.

Undernourished patients may show a shortened $t_{1/2}$ (e.g. antipyrine). The hepatic elimination of drugs with low clearance (due to strong protein binding) can be corrected by taking the extent of binding into consideration. Protein binding of many drugs is reduced in liver disease and this should be taken into account in calculating C_u, so that the change in metabolism can be recognized (e.g. valproic acid, brotizolam and nitrazepam).

The change in pharmacokinetics in acute hepatitis (e.g. tolbutamide, phenytoin) appears to be reversible and control values are reached after the patient recovers from the disease. Investigations with pethidine in acute and recovery phases showed an altered and normalising clearance respectively. Similarly the impaired elimination of diazepam has gradually reached normal value as clinical laboratory parameters such as bilirubin, transaminases and serum albumin of the patients improved.

Elimination of numerous substances, which are biotransformed through oxidative phase-I reaction, is delayed in patients with impaired liver function. In contrast to this glucuronidation (phase-II reaction) does not seem to be affected as observed in case of many drugs (e.g. lorazepam, oxazepam, temapezam, phenprocoumon, carprofen) with the exception of zomepirac. In case of diminished elimination through altered metabolism the dose should be accordingly reduced (Table 9).

Age influences not only the relative and absolute size of the liver but also its activity and capacity to synthesize the metabolising enzymes. In newborns the elimination as a rule is very slow, whereas in infants and adolescents the metabolic activity is even greater than in adults. For example, CL of theophylline in children is 87 mL/h/kg and adults 57 mL/h/kg. In geriatric patients the elimination of some drugs (e.g. chlordiazepoxide, lidocaine) has been found to be slower whereas for others like phenytoin it is faster. Half-life of the model drug antipyrine is slightly prolonged in older subjects but the difference is negligible if smoking habits or vitamin deficiency are taken into consideration.

While conducting age-studies, one must pay attention to the fact whether the aged persons under investigation are of normal health or possibly suffering from different diseases (probably taking many drugs!). Similarly whether the change in $t_{1/2}$ is due to altered V or CL should be differentiated. Diazepam for example shows a 2 to 3 times prolongation in older subjects as a result of increased V_{ss} and V_p. On the other hand the elimination of nitrazepam is affected only in immobilized old patients but not in healthy elderly.

Enzymatic biotransformation capacity of liver is genetically determined. Identical twins in contrast to heterozygous twins show an identical $t_{1/2}$. For drugs which are predominantly acetylated (e.g. isoniazid, some sulfonamides, dapsone) two genetic polymorphisms can be identified (slow and rapid acetylators). Similar polymorphism is also observed in populations (extensive and

Table 9. Drugs, whose elimination is delayed in patients with reduced liver function following single dose administration

Drug	Control value		In patients with reduced liver function	
	$t_{1/2}$ (h)	CL (ml/min)	$t_{1/2}$ (h)	CL (ml/min)
Amobarbital	21	92	39	41
Antipyrine	12.0	50	30	20
Brotizolam	6.9	64 (612)[a]	12.8	45 (380)[a]
Chlordiazepoxide	7–19	15	35–100	7
Clindamycin	3.4	–	4.5	–
Desmethyldiazepam	50.9	11.3	108.2	4.6
Diazepam	46.6	26.6	105.6	13.8
Hexobarbital	–	260	–	105
Isoniazid	3.2	–	6.7	–
Lidocaine	1.8	703	4.9	419
Meprobamate	12.6	–	24.3	–
Nitrazepam	31	63 (427)[a]	31	59 (320)[a]
Pethidine	3.3	1300	7.0	655
Paracetamol	2.9	–	7.2	–
Phenobarbital	86	–	104	–
Phenylbutazone	78	–	100	–
Propranolol	2.9	920	20.9	364
Rifampicin	2.8	–	5.4	
Theophyllin	9.2	58	30.0	27
Valproic acid	12.2	7.8	18.9	8.9

[a] Value in brackets is CL_R.

poor metabolisers) with respect to oxidative metabolism of drugs (e.g. sparteine, debrisoquine, mephenytoin).

Living habits and environment can also influence the metabolic activity. For example $t_{1/2}$ of many drugs can be reduced in smokers by one fourth of the normal value and elimination of phenacetin shows dependence on the nature of diet (normal or fried food).

4.4 Presystemic elimination and bioavailability

Following oral administration drugs are often eliminated to a certain degree before they reach systemic circulation. This effect is hence called "first pass-effect" and mostly liver is responsible for this presystemic elimination. Blood, with absorbed drug reaches liver via portal vein and hepatic artery, where biotransformation of the drug takes place by suitable enzymes. These different metabolic reactions are best characterized by intrinsic clearance (see also Fig. 7).

$$CL_{int} = D(p.o.)/AUC = v_{max}/K_m = Q_H \cdot E/(1-E) \tag{88}$$

if the bioavailability of the drug is known, then

$$CL = F \cdot D(\text{p.o.})/AUC \tag{66}$$

from equations (66; see page 39) and (88) and from the relationship $CL = Q_H \cdot E$

$$CL/F = CL_{int} = Q_u \cdot E/F = Q_H \cdot E/(1-E) \tag{89}$$

by solving the equation (52)

$$E = CL_{int}/Q_H + CL_{int} \tag{90}$$

A definite amount of drug corresponding to the extraction ratio E, reaches systemic circulation and bioavailability can be expressed as

$$F = 1 - E \tag{91}$$

The above described equations are based on linear kinetics where the plasma concentrations are dose dependent. However, some drugs show a dose dependent first pass-effect (e.g. propranolol, metoprolol, lorcainide, phenacetin) due to the saturation of liver enzymes.

Model problem 13

The plasma clearance (CL) and renal clearance (Cl_R) of famotidine in a healthy subject to be 305 ml/min and 190 ml/min respectively. Assuming a hepatic plasma flow of 800 ml/min calculate the theoretical systemic bioavailability of famotidine.

Solution:

$CL_H = CL - CL_R = 305 - 190 = 115$ mL/min

$Q_H = 800$ mL/min

$E = CL_H/Q_H = 115/800 = 0.14$

$F = 1 - E = 0.86$ (or) 86%

Presystemic elimination may also take place in the gastrointestinal tract and the intestinal clearance is dependent on the mesenteric blood flow, intrinsic clearance of the tissue and the extent of drug-tissue binding.

In adition to these factors, permeability and surface area also play a considerable role. β-Methyldigoxin is only 8% metabolised following i.v. administration whereas about 20% is presystematically extracted following oral administration. The role of intestinal wall and the bowel contents is not yet clear. L-Dopa is not metabolised by liver, however, it undergoes a significant presystemic elimination through acid hydrolysis as well as intestinal bacterial metabolism. The preabsorptive elimination is dependent upon the condition of intestinal flora which decides the nature of reaction (e.g. hydrolysis, reduction, cleavage).

Following i.v. administration or inhalation the drug enters lungs before it reaches systemic circulation. Various metabolic reactions of amines, peptides, fatty acids, nucleotides and steroids take place in lungs (e.g. noradrenaline but not adrenaline inactivation, conversion of angiotensin I to active form II, inactivation of isoproterenol to 3-O-methylisoproterenol before absorption).

Presystemic elimination is particularly notable for drugs with high clearance (Table 10) as it could greatly affect their bioavailability. For these drugs the oral dose has to be higher than the i.v. dose to produce identical response.

Biovailability of a drug is dependent on the formulation. It is not an absolute or fixed value for any given drug as it may be influenced by the adjuvants used in the formulation. It is defined (by American FDA) as "the rate and extent to which the active drug ingredient or therapeutic moiety is absorbed from a drug product and becomes available at the site of drug action". The term "bioequivalence" is often used when two drug products containing the same drug have same bioavailability. Bioequivalence of different formulations can be definitely expressed only when bioavailability of these formulations has been determined. It should not be ignored that bioavailability is an expression which includes both rate and amount (extent) of drug absorption. From plasma concentration-time profile it is possible to obtain the parameters C_{max}, t_{max} and AUC. The bioavailability is usually determined by estimating AUC or cumulative amount excreted in urine or pharmacological effect.

Table 10. Drugs with presystemic elimination

Substance	Gastro-intestinal	Hepatic	Remarks
Acetylsalicylic acid	+	+	Dose dependent
5-Aminosalicylic acid	+	+	Dose dependent
L-Dopa	+		Dose dependent
Estradiol, Estriol	+	+	Jejunum portion
Flurazepam, Flunitrazepam	+	+	
Hydralazine		+	
Impiramine		+	
Isoproterenol	+	+	Metabolism in lungs
Isosorbide dinitrate		+	
Lidocaine		+	
Lorcainide		+	Dose dependent
Medazepam		+	
Methyldigoxin	+		
Metoprolol, Oxprenolol		+	Dose dependent
Midazolam		+	Dose dependent
Nitroglycerine		+	
Norfenefrine		+	
Nortriptyline		+	
Pentazocine		+	
Pethidine		+	
Phenacetin		+	Dose dependent
Propoxyphene		+	Dose dependent
Propranolol, Alprenolol		+	Dose dependent
Salicylamide	+	+	Dose dependent
Verapamil		+	

The absolute (simultaneous i.v. administration is necessary) or relative (standard and reference substances) bioavailability is mostly determined following single dose administration. This, however, does not permit in each case extrapolation to clinical situation where the drug is repeatedly administered.

The bioavailability of drugs (with hepatic clearance > 1000 ml/min) which exhibit capacity limited first pass-effect under steady state conditions, is higher during therapy involving repeated administration than following a single dose administration (e.g. lorcainide, phenacetin).

Bioavailability studies are often conducted in a crossover design to minimize the interindividual variations, particularly when the number of the subjects is small. For the bioequivalence studies to be statistically meaningful they should be conducted at least in 10 subjects (better in 12–16 subjects). It is equally important to obtain sufficient plasma concentration or pharmacological effect measurements. A relatively new technique called "stable isotope technique (SIT)" is often employed in pharmacokinetic studies. The drug is administered along with its labelled counterpart (containing a stable isotope element such as ^{14}C or deuterium). By simultaneously measuring both substances under identical experimental conditions the intraindividual variation (even if the number of subjects is small) is reduced. It is possible to study with the help of SIT only when the synthesis and analytical (mass spectrometry) methods are feasible. This method is particularly useful for drugs with high clearance (e.g. Ca-antagonists, β-blockers) whose elimination is mainly dependent on the perfusion of liver which shows considerable day to day fluctuations.

The bioavailability F is not same as the fraction absorbed, f_a of orally administered drug because the amount absorbed may partly undergo presystematic elimination (f_{fp}). Thus bioavailability, F equals $f_a \cdot f_{fp}$. Under the assumption that the areas under plasma concentration-time curves are proportinal to the dose (AUC$\sim$D), the ratio of AUCs following oral or other extravascular route and i.v. administration is defined as bioavailability (Fig. 8). It is usually expressed as percentage.

$$F = (D(i.v.) \cdot AUC(p.o.)/D(p.o.) \cdot AUC(i.v.)) \cdot 100 \quad (92)$$

where the areas are calculated using the trapezoidal method (see page 8). It is also possible to determine the bioavailability from urinary excretion data. The equation which is employed for this purpose is as follows.

$$F = (A_e^\infty(p.o.) \cdot D(i.v.)/A_e^\infty(i.v.) \cdot D(p.o.)) \cdot 100. \quad (93)$$

For calculating A_e^∞ the urine is preferably collected at least for 4 half-lives.

Determination of bioavailability often explains the reason for variability in drug action. It has been shown earlier that some drugs (e.g. digoxin, phenytoin) exhibit variable effect following administration of therapeutic doses. Determination of plasma concentrations reveal that optimum concentrations are not reached due to low absorption. Bioavailability of digoxin preparations for example varies in healthy subjects between 60–90%. The variability in bioavailability is considerably large (Table 11) because of the differences in biological factors such as gastric emptying, blood flow to g.i. tract or first

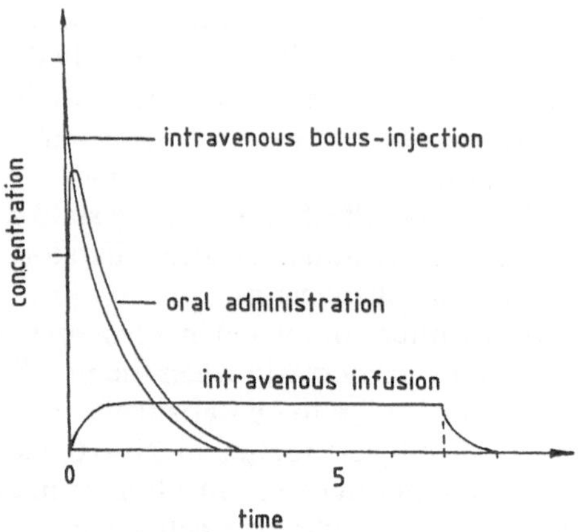

Fig. 8. Dost's rule of corresponding areas: The areas under time-plasma concentration curves is unchanged following i.v. bolus, i.v. infusion, or oral administration (with complete bioavailability) of a drug provided the dose administered is the same

Table 11. Factors, which can influence bioavailability

Pharmaceutical	Physiological
Particle size, solubility, crystal form, polymorphism, solvent system, formulation adjuvants, type of dosage form, manufacturing method	Age, sex, general state of health, time of administration, gastric emptying, intestinal motility, nutritients, disease, presystemic elimination

pass-effect. In patients the variability is even larger because of altered volume of distribution or protein binding. Similarly nutrients and co-administered drugs may alter absorption through interaction. However, the significance of bioavailability might be limited sometimes as it is not always possible to correlate plasma concentrations to the drug effect.

Following oral administration of high clearance drugs in patients with liver disease a considerable portion of absorbed dose bypasses the liver due to intra- and/or extra-hepatic shunts and thereby escapes metabolism during the first passage. This may result in a great increase in bioavailability (nearly 3 to 5 times) as observed in case of drugs like labetalol, lidocaine or verapamil. Such drugs therefore pose considerable risk in patients with reduced liver function and in such situations their dosage should be correspondingly reduced.

Model problem 14

Determine the absolute oral bioavailability of the new drug from the data given in model problems 1 (see page 5) and 4 (see page 21).

Solution:

$$D(i.v.) = D(p.o.) = 500\ mg = 500{,}000\ \mu g$$

$$AUC(i.v.) = 180\ \mu g \cdot h/mL;\quad AUC(p.o.) = 68.1\ \mu g/mL$$

$$F = [D(i.v.) \times AUC(p.o.)/D(p.o.) \times AUC(i.v.)] \times 100$$

$$= [500{,}000 \times 68.1/500{,}000 \times 180] \times 100 = 37.8\%$$

4.5 Other elimination processes

Next to renal and hepatic elimination, pulmonary elimination plays an important role (e.g. volatile anaesthetics). Some drugs which are not absorbed through gastrointestinal tract are formulated to produce a local effect (e.g. streptomycin, neomycin). These drugs are excreted in feces either unchanged or metabolized (by bacteria).

It may also be noticed in case of certain drugs that a definite percentage of administered dose is excreted into intestines through bile either unchanged or mostly in the form of glucuronide. Sometimes the glucuronide may be hydrolysed in the intestines by bacteria and the liberated free drug is reabsorbed. The reabsorbed drug is again converted into glucuronide in the liver and reexcreted into the intestines. This enterohepatic circulation can lead to extended drug action. Such drugs which are essentially excreted through bile may be conveniently administered in diseases involving biliary tract so that high drug concentrations are maintained in situ for longer periods. In certain intoxications (e.g. digitoxin) it is possible to trap part of the excreted dose in the intestines by administration of adsorbents like activated charcoal or cholestyramine.

Drugs which are excreted through bile by active and capacity limited secretion have molecular weight above 500 and often possess a strongly polar group. These prerequisits are managed by coupling with glucuronic acid, which increases the M.W. by about 200 and significantly enhances the polarity.

4.6 Kinetics of metabolism

It was already mentioned in the previous sections that the metabolites of some drugs are partly active (see Table 6). These metabolites may often produce toxic effects (e.g. halothane, glutethimide) or may interfere with the action of parent substance or other drugs. Elimination of metabolite is in general dependent on its own formation because its elimination begins as soon as it is formed. In such an instance the fall in concentration of parent drug and its metabolite takes place parallel to each other with the same $t_{1/2}$ and the plasma concentration-time profile of the metabolite lies under that of the parent drug (e.g. tolbutamide-hydroxytolbutamide). A metabolite can accumulate in the body when its elimination takes place very slowly. Only in such an instance the fall in concentration is controlled through its own $t_{1/2}$ and the plasma concentration curve of metabolite lies above the curve of the drug (e.g. glutethimide – 4-hydroxy glutethimide, diazepam – desmethyldiazepam). From areas under the respective curves one can compute clearances of metabolite (M) and parent compound (P).

The fraction of drug which has undergone metabolism is given by

$$AUC_M/AUC_P = f_M \cdot (CL_P/CL_M)\,. \qquad (94)$$

This important relationship makes the calculation of metabolite clearance simple (when f_M is equal to 1 and when only one metabolite is formed).

The fraction of a dose of P that is metabolised to M can be determined as following:

$$f_M = (AUC_{M(P)}/D_P)/(AUC_{M(M)}/D_M) \qquad (94\,a)$$

where $AUC_{M(P)}$ and $AUC_{M(M)}$ refer to the AUC of the metabolite following the dosing of parent compount (D_P) or the metabolite (D_M) itself.

Part II

Pharmacokinetic principles and their clinical significance

1 Introduction

The first part of this book enables the reader to be familiarized with basic concepts of pharmacokinetics (*A*bsorption, *D*istribution, *M*etabolism and *E*xcretion – ADME) following single dose administration. In this part these principles are applied to clinically relevant situations, namely, multiple or (sub) chronic administration. In day to day practice besides acute drug response, often a longer duration of action is desired. This situation needs the understanding of changes in pharmacokinetics of drugs upon repeated administration, and the dosage regimen has to be accordingly adjusted for achieving uniform therapeutic levels for desired period of time.

2 Multiple dosing

The basic mathematical relationships applicable to single dose administration kinetics are also valid (with slight modifications) for multiple dose kinetics. In multiple dose therapy the ultimate purpose is to achieve a steady drug effect or response with minimum side effects. As mentioned before, this can be achieved in most cases by maintaining the plasma concentrations in therapeutic range for required number of hours or days. This may be considered as a general rule with an exception of nitrates, in which case the concentrations during the interval between two doses (called "dosing interval") should fall below a critical threshold level, such that tolerance does not develop.

A drug is commonly administered in fixed doses at constant intervals of time so that the amount lost through elimination is replaced after each dose. This kind of administration is associated with some fluctuations in drug concentrations in the body followed by a steady state condition. Time required for the steady state concentrations to reach can be exactly estimated.

2.1 Infusion

In view of safety (e.g. aminoglycosides, methotrexate) and/or pharmacokinetic reasons (e.g. lidocaine, nitroprusside, dopamine) some intravenously administered drugs are given as short infusion instead of bolus. This is to avoid the occurrence of a toxic peak or to compensate the drug loss due to quick elimination and to maintain a steady therapeutic concentration. Following a constant infusion rate R_0 (mass per unit time), the concentrations do not rise in a linear fashion but show an exponential behaviour as elimination also takes place simultaneously. The curve becomes asymptotic until a steady state concentration, C^{ss} is reached (see Fig. 9). From this time point onwards the concentration remains constant as a result of simultaneous invasion and elimination processes. When there is an interruption in the infusion, the plasma concentrations fall exponentially as in the case of i.v. bolus administration (Fig. 9). The time required to reach the steady state condition can be determined based on terminal half-life ($t_{1/2}$) of the drug.

The significance of $t_{1/2}$ with respect to accumulation and elimination is given in Table 12. After a time interval equivalent to one half-life, 50% of the drug is eliminated and the concentration reaches only 50% of C^{ss}. It needs about 4 to 5 elimination half-lives to reach 94–97% of C^{ss} ($3.3 \times t_{1/2}$ for 90% of C^{ss}). It is often desirable to shorten this time gap and reach C^{ss} quickly by administration of an i.v. loading bolus at the beginning of the infusion (Table 12).

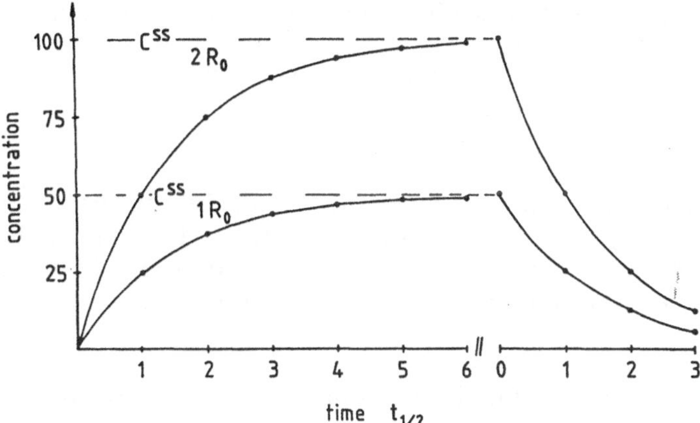

Fig. 9. Schematic representation of change in concentration during an i.v. infusion with the infusion rate (dose) 1 R_0 and doubled infusion rate 2 R_0. C^{ss} is reached after 5–6 elimination half-lives. The concentration fall, following interruption of the infusion shows the same exponential fall as after an i.v. bolus

Table 12. Duration of an infusion (or repeated administration), % of C^{ss} reached, drug eliminated and still in the body

Duration (times $t_{1/2}$)	Percent C^{ss} reached	After completion of infusion	
		Percent eliminated	Percent still in the body
1	50	50	50
2	75	75	25
3	87.5	87.5	12.5
4	93.8	93.8	6.2
5	96.9	96.9	3.1
6	98.4	98.4	1.6
7	99.2	99.2	0.8

It is possible to judge the toxic or therapeutic effect of administered dose only after 4 to 5 $t_{1/2}$ (taking the new C^{ss} into consideration). The height of plateau (C^{ss}) is determined by the rate of infusion R_0. The formulae for determination of C^{ss} for different compartment models are as follows

one compartment	two compartment	multi-compartment
$C^{ss} = R_0/k \cdot V$	$C^{ss} = R_0/k_{10} \cdot V_p$	$C^{ss} = R_0/\lambda_z \cdot V_z$
		$= R_0/CL$ (95)

The amount of drug in the body is directly proportional to the rate of infusion (R_0). Increasing the speed of infusion will result in a proportional increase in C^{ss} (see Fig. 9). On the other hand, smaller volume of distribution (V_p or V_z) and slower elimination (k or CL) will increase C^{ss}. Under steady state condition, the rate of infusion (R_0) and of elimination ($k \cdot C^{ss} \cdot V$) are balanced as shown in the equation (96).

$$R_0 = k \cdot V \cdot C^{ss} = CL \cdot C^{ss} \tag{96}$$

The steady state condition can be reached rapidly by administration of an i.v. bolus (or slow injection) before starting the infusion. This initial dose is adjusted depending on the volume of distribution of the drug and the desired plasma concentration. Rewriting the above equation yields

$$C^{ss} \cdot V = R_0/k \tag{97}$$

In steady state the amount of drug in the body must be exactly equal to DL (loading dose).

$$DL = C^{ss} \cdot V \quad \text{or} \quad DL = R_0/k \tag{98}$$

For the estimation of initial dose it is necessary to know the elimination constant and the rate of infusion which depend upon the individual patient clearance and the desired steady state concentration.

Model problem 15

The elimination rate constant of a drug which was infused at a rate of 200 μg/min was 0.35 h^{-1}. If the apparent volume of distribution of the drug is 20 L and assuming open 1-compartment model estimate the steady state concentration. What is the loading dose to be administered to achieve this concentration rapidly.

Solution:

$$k = 0.35\ h^{-1};\quad V = 20\ L;\quad R_0 = 200\ \mu g/min$$

$$C^{ss} = R_0/k \cdot V = (200 \times 60)/(0.35 \times 20{,}000)$$
$$= 1.71\ \mu g/mL$$

$$DL = C^{ss} \cdot V$$
$$= 1.71 \times 20{,}000$$
$$= 34{,}200\ \mu g \quad \text{(or)} \quad 34.2\ mg.$$

2.2 Repeated dose administration

In daily practice most of the drugs are administered not once but repeatedly to achieve a longer duration of action. A constant dose administered at definite time intervals (dosage interval = τ) is comparable to an intermittent infusion. In principle the same rules are applicable as in case of infusion and the steady state concentrations are achieved in 4 to 5 half-lives but the concentrations during a dosing interval fluctuate around a definite average concentration (C^{ss}_{av}).

Shortly after oral administration the peak that appears is the highest concentration (C^{ss}_{max}) and the concentration before the next dose is the lowest (C^{ss}_{min}), known as "trough".

Similarly following parenteral administration (see Fig. 10) as in case of i.v. infusion the maximum concentration C^{ss}_{max} which is achieved after 5 $t_{1/2}$ depends on the dose D administered or the fraction of the dose which is bioavailable (F = 1 in case of i.v. administration or complete bioavailability), volume of distribution, elimination rate and dosing interval.

one compartment	multi compartment	
$C^{ss}_{av} = F \cdot D/k \cdot V$	$C^{ss}_{av} = F \cdot D/\lambda_z V_z$	
$= F \cdot D/CL \cdot \tau$	$= F \cdot D/CL \cdot \tau$	(99)

As it can be seen from the above equations that C^{ss}_{av} is model independent but it is directly proportional to the dose and inverse proportional to the total clearance and dosing interval. A reduction in clearance or a shorter dosing interval result in increased C^{ss}_{av}. The physician can choose a suitable "dosing rate (D/τ)" depending on the desired therapeutic concentration (C^{ss}_{av}) and this rate should of course be in accordance with individual clearance. It is obvious from these observations that L C is the most important parameter from patient's side which determines C^{ss}_{av} (Fig. 10).

The longer the interval between two individual doses the greater will be the fluctuations in concentrations ($C^{ss}_{max} - C^{ss}_{min}$) around the average concentration

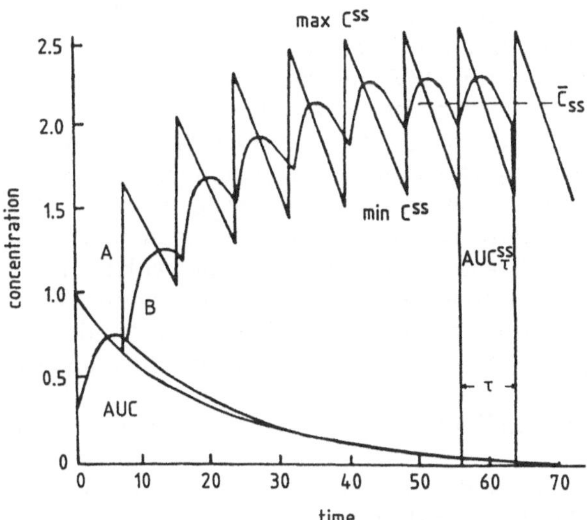

Fig. 10. Concentration changes following repeated i.v. (*curve A*) and repeated oral (*curve B*) administration of the same dose of drug. After a time period (equivalent to 5–6 $t_{1/2}$), the mean steady state concentration (C^{ss}_{av}), which fluctuates during the dosing interval (τ), between maximum and minimum C^{ss}), is reached. The area under the curve during the dosing interval (AUC^{ss}_{τ}) is equal to the AUC after a single dose (AUC)

C^{ss}_{av}. C^{ss}_{av} is calculated taking the logarithmic mean instead of arithmetic mean of C^{ss}_{max} and C^{ss}_{min} as given below

$$C^{ss}_{av} = (C^{ss}_{max} - C^{ss}_{min}) / \ln(C^{ss}_{max}/C^{ss}_{min}) \quad (100)$$

Both these extreme values following multiple administration in case of one compartment model can be calculated from the following equations

(a) i.v. administration

$$C^{ss}_{max} = (D/V)/1 - e^{-k \cdot \tau} \qquad C^{ss}_{min} = ((D/V)/1 - e^{-k \cdot \tau}) \cdot e^{-k \cdot \tau} = C^{ss}_{max} \cdot e^{-k \cdot \tau} \quad (101)$$

(b) In case of oral administration when the rate of absorption is assumed to be much larger than the rate of elimination and if the bioavailability (F) is known

$$C^{ss}_{max} = F \cdot D/V(1 - e^{-k \cdot \tau}) \quad (102)$$

$$C^{ss}_{min} = (F \cdot D \cdot e^{-k \cdot \tau})/V(1 - e^{-k \cdot \tau}) \quad (103)$$

The same equation can be used for drugs whose pharmacokinetics are better described by two compartment model and when the next dosing definitely follows after the distribution phase ($\tau > 3/\lambda_1$) then the equation for C^{ss}_{min} is as follows

$$C^{ss}_{min} = (F \cdot D \cdot e^{-\lambda_z \cdot \tau})/V(1 - e^{-\lambda_z \cdot \tau}) \quad (104)$$

It is therefore evident that the distribution phase (necessary for describing the disposition following a single dose administration with the help of λ_1) can be neglected. The two compartment model kinetics following single dose approach the one compartment model upon multiple administration.

To reduce the magnitude of fluctuations in maximum and minimum steady state concentrations around C^{ss}_{av} and consequently to avoid toxicity or ineffectiveness, it is better to administer relatively smaller doses in shorter intervals. For example, a 200 mg/6 h regimen is better than 400 mg/12 h regimen. In practice, to keep these variations within certain limits, τ should not be longer than $t_{1/2}$. The fluctuations are proportional to the ratio $\tau/t_{1/2}$ and they are reduced through retarded absorption. If $t_{1/2}$ is chosen to be the dosing interval, then C^{ss}_{min} will be half of C^{ss}_{max} and as a result, drugs with $t_{1/2}$ more than 36 h (e.g. digoxin, phenobarbital) can be administered only once daily. The dosing interval should be increased or better the dosage decreased under reduced clearance conditions (e.g. renal or hepatic insufficiency) as there is an increase in C^{ss}_{av} (see page 43).

Under normal conditions there are two possibilities for achieving C^{ss} (see also Fig. 11).

(1) The maintenance dose is administered after a recommended time lapse. It takes about 4 to 5 $t_{1/2}$ for the C^{ss}_{av} to be reached (e.g. digoxin, which has a $t_{1/2}$ of about 36 h takes nearly a week for the equilibrium to be reached).

(2) A higher initial dose has to be administered to achieve an early steady state condition (for quicker onset of action). The stated maintenance is administered subsequently at recommended intervals of time.

The loading (DL) and maintenance dose ($DM = D/\tau$) are calculated with known V and CL values.

Example for dosage calculation:

	digoxin	theophylline
$DL = C^{ss} \cdot V$	1.5 µg/L × 600 L = 0.9 mg	10 mg/L × 0.35 L = 350 mg
$DM = C^{ss} \cdot CL$	1.5 µg/L × 8 L/h = 12 µg/h = 0.29 mg/day	10 mg/L × 4 L/h = 40 mg/h = 960 mg/day

For digoxin and theophylline the therapeutically "desired" concentrations are taken as 1.5 µg/L and 10 mg/L respectively.

When the system is in a steady state, AUC following administration of maintenance dose during the dosing interval must be equal to AUC following single dose administration so that the dose independent (linear) kinetics can be applied (see Fig. 10; Fig. 11). A significant difference between the theoretically (using equation 99) calculated and the experimentally measured values of C^{ss}

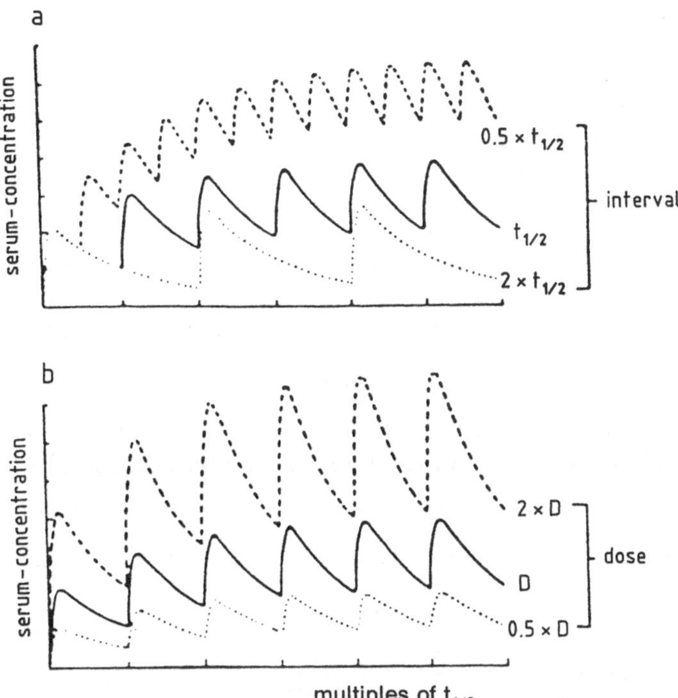

Fig. 11 a, b. a The influence of change in dosing interval on the steady state profile of a drug at a given dose D. **b** The influence of change in dose on the steady state profile at a constant dosing interval

indicates that the pharmacokinetics (V, CL and F) of the drug are changing upon multiple administration and non-linear kinetics have to be assumed.

As in case of single dose administration, the total clearance can be calculated also in steady state condition using AUC during dosing interval

$$CL = F \cdot D/AUC_{\tau}^{ss} \tag{105}$$

The renal clearance can be calculated by measuring the amount of unchanged drug excreted in urine (Ae_{τ}) and the corresponding AUC during the period

$$CL_R = Ae_{\tau}/AUC_{\tau}^{ss} \tag{106}$$

The mean steady state concentration can be determined once AUC_{τ}^{ss} is known

$$C_{av}^{ss} = AUC_{\tau}^{ss}/\tau \tag{107}$$

Many fixed drug combinations of two or more substances in a single formulation are not meaningful on pharmacokinetic grounds. As these combinations often consist of drugs with different $t_{1/2}$ and CL values, it is not possible to simultaneously achieve therapeutic concentrations for all components by choosing a single and arbitrary dosing interval. To avoid such discrepancies it is advisable to administer them separately.

2.3 Accumulation

Repeated or multiple administration may often lead to drug accumulation in the body. Accumulation is not a specific property of only some drugs but it is always noticed following administration of a new dose while a portion of the previously administered dose is still in the body. When a gap of 4 to 5 $t_{1/2}$ exists between two doses in multiple administration therapy, over 98% of the previous dose is eliminated before a new dose is administered and accumulation is avoided. However, such an approach is not desired as it results in longer periods of ineffective concentrations. The extent of accumulation is therefore dependent on the ratio between τ and $t_{1/2}$, which is expressed as factor (relative dosing interval)

$$\varepsilon = \tau/t_{1/2}\,. \tag{108}$$

Analogous to steady state concentrations at equilibrium the amount of drug in the body following a single dose administration may be expressed as

$$A_{max} = D/(1 - e^{-k/\tau}) = D/(1 - 2^{-\varepsilon}) \tag{109}$$

The accumulated amount after a dosing interval, before the next dose is administered is

$$A_{min} = A_{max} - D = D \cdot (1/1 - 2^{-\varepsilon} - 1) \tag{110}$$

In case of digitoxin ($t_{1/2} = 120$ h) for example, when administered once daily ($\tau = 24$ h) has factor $\varepsilon = 0.2$. From Table 13

$$A_{max} = D/(1 - 2^{-0.2}) = D/(1 - 0.871) = D \times 7.73$$

$$A_{min} = D \times (7.73 - 1) = D \times 6.73$$

It is obvious that in digitalization the steady state maximum and minimum amounts in the body are respectively by a factor 7.7 and 6.7 higher than the amounts following a single dose administration. Accumulation may be rapidly realized by administering an initial loading dose equivalent to the sum of A_{min} and maintenance dose (DM), which in our present example is equal to 0.1 mg/die. Then

$$DL = DM + A_{min} = 0.1\ mg + D \cdot 6.73$$
$$= 0.1 + 0.1 \times 6.73 = 0.77\ mg$$

Loading dose can also be calculated from V and C_{av}^{ss} (in the present example, they are 37.5 L and 20 μg/L respectively) for comparison.

$$DL = C_{av}^{ss} \cdot V = 20 \times 37.5 = 0.75\ mg$$

which gives nearly the same result.

The mathematical relationship $1/(1 - e^{\lambda_z \cdot \tau}) = 1/(1 - 2^{-\varepsilon})$ is defined (see equation 109) as accumulation factor R_K (see Table 13). When $\tau = t_{1/2}$ the R_K value is 2.0 which can be considered as a kind of standard. The value of R_K is larger than 2.0 when τ is smaller than $t_{1/2}$ (e.g. $R_K = 3.4$ when $\tau = 0.5 \cdot t_{1/2}$) and it is less than 2.0 when τ is larger than $t_{1/2}$ (e.g. $R_K = 1.33$ when $\tau = 2 \cdot t_{1/2}$). With the help of this factor DL can be calculated simply from the equation

$$DL = R_K \cdot DM \tag{111}$$

All these relationships are valid only for i.v. administration, however, they can also be used in case of p.o. administration provided it is surely known that for the drug in question the absorption is essentially faster than the elimination (Table 13).

Table 13. Dependence of accumulation factor (R_K) on the relative dosing interval (τ)

$\varepsilon = \tau/t_{1/2}$	$2^{-\varepsilon}$	R_K	$\varepsilon = \tau/t_{1/2}$	$2^{-\varepsilon}$	R_K
0.01	0.993	145	0.8	0.574	2.34
0.05	0.966	29.4	0.9	0.536	2.15
0.1	0.933	14.9	1.0	0.50	2.0
0.2	0.871	7.72			
0.3	0.812	5.32	2.0	0.250	1.33
0.4	0.758	4.12	3.0	0.125	1.14
0.5	0.707	3.44	4.0	0.063	1.07
0.6	0.660	2.93	5.0	0.031	1.03
0.7	0.616	2.6			

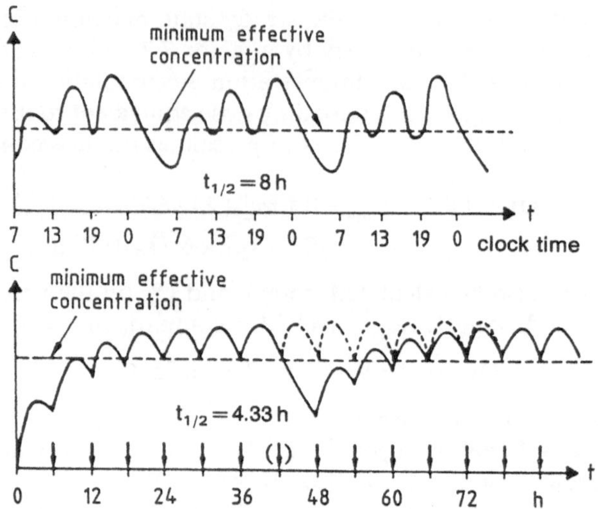

Fig. 12. Schematic representation of the changes in plasma concentration profiles, above: irregular dosing (7.00, 13.00 and 19.00 hrs), below: the maintenance dose has been "forgotten" once

It is to be further considered that in practice it is difficult to expect a constant and regular dosing to be maintained by the patient. It is possible that often some doses are skipped. The consequences of such irregularities (influencing the plasma concentration-time profile) are schematically depicted in Figure 12.

3 Drug interactions

Most patients receive more than one drug at a time, which can often lead to unexpected or even adverse effects. These effects are often due to interactions of drugs. Drug–drug interactions may be pharmacologically synergistic or antagonistic. The interaction between two substances can take place either outside the body (incompatibilities) or within the body (pharmacodynamic or -kinetic interactions). This section deals only with the latter.

About 7% of the undesirable effects in therapy are due to drug interactions and their incidence increases exponentially with the number of drugs administered simultaneously. The number of theoretical possibilities N may be mathematically expressed as

$$N = (\text{number of drugs})!/2!\,(\text{number of drugs} - 2)! \qquad (112)$$

Administration of 7 drugs simultaneously for example may result in about $(7!/2! \times 5!) = 21$ possible interactions.

3.1 Absorption interactions

Drugs which alter pH and motility of gastrointestinal tract can influence the rate and the extent of absorption of the co-administered drug. H_2-receptor antagonists by inhibiting gastric acid secretion may result in altered absorption of other drugs which are administered simultaneously (e.g. cimetidine hinders the absorption of ketaconazole). On the other hand, in the treatment of peptic ulcer simultaneous administration of antacids may reduce the absorption of a H_2-receptor antagonist, which can be avoided by administering these two drugs with an interval of 2 h.

Anticholinergic agents (e.g. atropine) and opiates (e.g. morphine, codeine) by prolonging the gastric emptying time, may delay the absorption of other drugs (e.g. propanthelin significantly reduces the absorption of paracetamol). Certain drugs like metoclopramide on the contrary, accelerate the absorption of alcohol and paracetamol by enhancing the gastric emptying rate.

The salts of multivalent metallic ions (Ca^{+2}, Mg^{+2}, Fe^{+2}, Al^{+3}) such as constituents of food and antacids form poorly absorbable complexes with drugs like tetracyclines. The ion exchange resin, cholestyramine which shows strong affinity to acidic drugs such as warfarin, aspirin and digitoxin forms complexes and hinders their absorption. Similarly the bioavailability of rifampicin is reduced to about 50% when administered along with PAS granules. The binding agents used in the manufacture of granules have been found to form poorly soluble complexes with rifampicin.

In patients with chronic inflammatory bowel diseases the extent of availability of 5-aminosalicylic acid (mesalazine) following reductive cleavage of the administered azo prodrug, sulfasalazine by colon bacteria is affected by diarrhoea which is a frequent symptom in these patients and simultaneous administration of antibiotics which influence the intestinal flora.

3.2 Distribution interactions

These interactions mostly arise from competition between two substances for the same protein binding sites in plasma and tissues. Changes in the action of drugs often occur under the following conditions. When

(a) the drug in question has a narrow therapeutic range
(b) there exists a relationship between free (unbound) drug concentration and effect
(c) the apparent volume of distribution is less than 2 L/kg
(d) the plasma protein binding is above 80% ($f_u < 0.2$) and
(e) the saturation of binding sites takes place in the normal therapeutic dose range.

Some drugs particularly amitryptiline, desimipramine, digitoxin, disopyramide, imipramine, nortriptyline, phenytoin, phenylbutazone, salicylic acid, tolbutamide, valproic acid and warfarin with the above characteristics often pose problems in therapy.

It was found through different experiments that the human serum albumin (HSA) has 3 binding sites. These sites which can be characterized by "markers" like diazepam, warfarin and digitoxin, are saturated beyond a particular concentration of the ligand (a drug or an endogenous substance). Competition between different ligands under physiological conditions leads to displacement interaction. Basically such interactions may be expected for drugs which show concentration dependent protein binding (e.g. disopyramide, phenylbutazone and salicylates). Some clinically relevant interactions include displacement of phenytoin by valproic acid, warfarin by phenylbutazone and valproic acid by salicylates.

In general, it can be stated that with reduced plasma protein binding the apparent volume of distribution increases because the distribution of greater part of drug into tissues (due to increased free fraction) takes place. The following relationship is applicable for apparent volume of distribution

$$V_{ss} = V_p + V_t \cdot (f_p/f_t) \tag{61}$$

From the above equation it is obvious that V_{ss} is dependent on plasma and tissue protein binding (see also page 36).

Clearance (CL) which depends on intrinsic clearance (CL_{int}), blood flow to the elimination organs (Q) and F (see page 49) is regarded as a very important parameter. In case of restrictive tpye of elimination (e.g. warfarin, phenytoin, diazepam) the unbound fraction (f_u) or protein binding determines CL and in such cases the steady state concentration (C_u^{ss}) is given by

$$C_u^{ss} = F \cdot D/CL_{int} \cdot \tau \tag{113}$$

It is evident that C_u^{ss} remains unaffected by changes in protein binding due to interactions. Hence it must be considered that the initial increase in C_u^{ss} is only short lived (see Fig. 13).

In contrast to the above observation the total concentration (C^{ss}, free + bound) is proportional to f_u or sensitive to changes in binding (see Fig. 13)

$$C^{ss} = F \cdot D/CL_{int} \cdot f_u \cdot \tau \tag{114}$$

In case of drugs which do not fall under "restrictive type of elimination" category (e.g. propranolol, lidocaine) the clearance is dependent on the blood flow to the elimination organs and the total concentration is not significantly affected by protein binding. This, however, is not applicable for C_u^{ss} ($= C^{ss} \cdot f_u$), which is proportionately altered by changes in f_u (extent of protein binding).

Due to difference in binding affinity to liver proteins the combination of antimalarials mepacrine and pamacrine (less strongly bound) may exhibit toxic side effects depending on sequence of administration. Another well known interaction is between quinidine and digoxin (see page 76) in which case the volume of distribution of the latter is altered by the former.

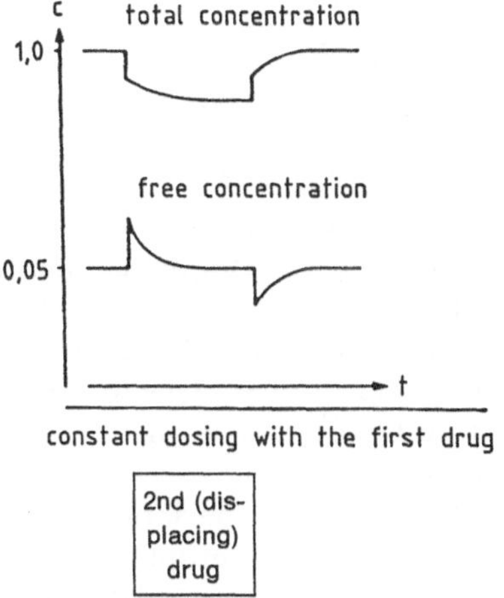

Fig. 13. The change in steady state plasma concentration profile of a drug, which is strongly protein bound and has a restricted clearance, upon administration of another drug which displaces it from the protein binding sites. A significant change in total (above) and unbound (below) drug concentration followed by a rapid establishment of new lower C^{ss} with the same C_u^{ss}, is observed

3.3 Elimination interactions

Many interactions take place at the hepatic level. These are usually accomplished through modifications in functional activity of microsomal enzymes which are either activated (induction) or inhibited. Smoking, chronic alcohol consumption in moderate doses, pesticides, barbiturates, anticonvulsants (particularly carbamazepine and phenytoin), rifampicin, glutethimide, chloralhydrate and phenylbutazone are well known inducers of liver microsomal enzyme systems. When drugs such as anticonvulsants, oral anticoagulants, digitoxin, antiarrhythmics and oral contraceptives are administerd along with an inducer, their effectiveness is reduced due to enhanced metabolism. As these enzymes are nonspecific, the metabolism of some endogenous substances such as steroid hormones (glucocorticoids, androgens, oestrogens, progesterones, cortisol etc.), bilirubin and vitamin D is likewise accelerated in presence of inducers. However, induction usually needs some time to develop and pretreatment with the inducers (usually a few days) is necessary. During induction, the protein synthesis in other words the enzyme content in liver increases and during competitive inhibition, the microsomal activity of cytochrome P450 system is reduced.

Monoaminooxidase (MAO) inhibitors act by blockade of metabolism of catecholamines (e.g. dopamine, tyramine, serotonine, noradrenaline, adrenaline). For this reason patients receiving MAO inhibitors should avoid taking food stuff containing tyramine (e.g. cheese, salt herrings, soy beans, meat, yeast extract, chicken livers). Administration of L-dopa also rises dopamine and noradrenaline levels and hence increases the risk of hypertension.

MAO inhibitors can prolong the hypoglycaemic effect of oral antidiabetic agents through interference with the normal adrenergic stimulus. Therefore, care should be taken while administering these agents in patients with diabetes. Administration of a MAO inhibitor and pethidine can produce excitation, profuse perspiration, rigidity, hypertension (probably also a fall in B.P.) and coma. The mechanism of this interaction is still not known.

Simultaneous administration of MAO inhibitors, particularly tranylocypromine along with a sympathomimetic amine such as amphetamine, ephedrine (included in numerous combinations), phenylephrine (in many formulations including nasal sprays) and phenylpropanolamine results in increased release and accumulation of noradrenaline. In addition, inhibition of metabolism of phenylephrine also takes place in presence of MAO inhibitors. Both these mechanisms result in hypertension, disturbances in cardiac rhythm, headache and fever (upto 43 °C).

Other known inhibitors are allopurinol and chloramphenicol. The metabolism of azathioprine and mercaptopurine is inhibited by allopurinol through xanthineoxidase blockade and that of dicumarol by chloramphenicol. H_2-receptor antagonists (e.g. cimetidine, ranitidine, famotidine) depending on chemical structure exhibit variable binding affinity for cytochrome P450. Cimetidine through a stronger affinity inhibits the metabolism of many drugs. Ranitidine has only a weak and famotidine has almost no affinity for this

Table 14. Cimetidine inhibits the hepatic elimination of:

Acenocoumarol	Desmethyldiazepam	Lidocaine	Quinidine
Alcohol	Diazepam	Metoprolol	Quinine
Alprazolam	Doxepine	Metronidazole	Salicylic acid
Antipyrine	Ethmozine	Nifedipine	Theobromine
Bromazepam	Femoxetine	Nitrazepam	Theophylline
Caffeine	5-Fluorouracil	Pefloxacine	Triamterene
Carbamazepam	Glibenclamide	Phenandione	Triazolam
Chlordiazepoxide	Gliclazide	Phenytoin	Trimazosine
Chlormethiazole	Imipramine	Procainamide	Valproic acid
Clobazam	Labetalol	Propranolol	Verapamil
			Warfarin

important coenzyme. Therefore, the interaction potential of these two drugs is much lower than that of cimetidine (Table 14).

Isoniazid, disulfiram, propranolol (also metoprolol to some extent), oral contraceptives and high, acute alcohol consumption may also inhibit the hepatic metabolism of diazepam, antipyrine and theophylline.

Elimination of the so called "high clearance" drugs (see page 49) is also determined by blood flow to the elimination organs. Propranolol by reducing (depending on dose) the cardiac output lowers the liver blood flow and this effect leads to reduction in its own clearance and that of other high clearance drugs (e.g. lidocaine).

Numerous interactions have been reported also in case of *renal elimination.* For example the amount of unchanged amphetamine excreted in acidic urine (pH 5) is more (60–70%) than in alkalized urine (10%). Similarly as mentioned earlier, the excretion of acidic drugs like salicylates and barbiturates can be enhanced by alkalization, which plays an important role in the management of poisoning by these agents.

As renal elimination of lithium, which takes place through glomerular filtration, is influenced by tubular reabsorption process, it is not wonder that the plasma concentrations of Li^+ can be affected by different diuretics through their influence on either of the two mechanisms. Acetazolamide and methylxanthine accelerate the excretion of Li^+ by impairing its tubular reabsorption. However, furosemide and thiazide diuretics result in elevated plasma concentrations of Li^+ by enhancing its tubular reabsorption (reducing Li^+ clearance by 25%). With the exception of acetylsalicylic acid, different non-steroidal antiphlogistic agents such as phenylbutazone, indomethacin and diclofenac significantly increase the plasma levels of Li^+ (intoxication risk!) by reducing its renal clearance.

Different acidic drugs like probenecid, acetylsalicylic acid, sulfonamides, furosemide and ethacrynic acid inhibit the renal elimination of penicillin through competitive blockade of proximal tubular active secretion. Similarly the secretion of basic drugs such as procainamide, N-acetylprocainamide, metformin and triamterene is inhibited by cimetidine and to a very low extent by ranitidine.

Table 15. Some clinically important drug interactions

Drug	Interferes with	Clinical observation
Amphotericin B	Digitalis glycosides	Hypokalemia/digitalis intoxication
Antacids (Ca^{+2}, Mg^{+2}, Al^{+3})	Tetracyclines	Reduced absorption
Antidiabetics	Anticoagulants	Hypoglycemia, reduced prothrombin time
Barbiturates, Glutethimide, Rifampicin	Anticoagulants and many other drugs	Accelerated metabolism
Cimetidine	Diazepam and many other drugs	Reduced metabolism/higher plasma levels (toxicity)
Cytostatic drugs	Digoxin	Impaired absorption
Disulfiram	Alcohol, Phenytoin, Warfarin	Reduced metabolism
Phenylbutazone	Anticoagulants, Antidiabetics, Phenytoin	Potentiation of drug action
Propranolol	Oral antidiabetics	Severe hypokalemia, increased blood pressure
Quinidine	Digoxin (Digitoxin?)	Increased plasma levels (toxicity!)
Salicylates	Anticoagulants	Reduction in prothrombin concentration, bleeding
Salicylates	Probenecid, Sulfinpyrazone	Inhibition of increased uric acid excretion
Salicylates	Methotrexate	Increased MTX levels (toxicity!)
Steroids (anabolic)	Anticoagulants	Increased bleeding

A complex interaction is noticed between quinidine and digoxin. It was observed in many investigations that quinidine increases the plasma levels of digoxin. It is well known that quinidine inhibits both renal (CL_R) and nonrenal (CL_{NR}) clearance of digoxin. In addition to this effect, changes in volume of distribution of digoxin might also take place. At the moment it is not clear whether the kinetics of digitoxin also are slightly influenced by quinidine.

Interaction between quinidine and digoxin has stimulated investigations on influence of different antiarrhythmic agents and Ca^{+2}-antagonists on kinetics of digoxin. It is interesting to note that verapamil, diltiazem and amiodarone are very similar to quinidine in affecting digoxin kinetics, whereas nifedipine, gallopamil, captopril and propafenone have a very mild influence. Disopyramide, mexilitine, prajmaline, lidoflazine and procainamide have no effect at all.

Different clinically important drug interactions are given in Table 15. The interaction potential of drugs can be estimated from their pharmacological or pharmacokinetic properties, provided the general principles and mechanisms are known. Animal and in vitro experiments can be helpful in predicting often these interactions.

4 Concentration – effect relationships

The ultimate purpose of drug therapy lies in utilization of the pharmacodynamic response i.e., the drug should produce desired biological effect at a specific site (organ or tissue) in the body, where it is required. It is relatively easier to determine the pharmacokinetic parameters based on drug concentrations in plasma or urine than to measure the pharmacodynamic or therapeutic responses, which very often involve methodical difficulties. B. B. Brodie (1945) stated that the drug effects are better correlated to plasma concentrations rather than administered dose. It is well known that for a given drug in each patient the plasma concentration–time profile is dependent on many exogenous as well as endogenous factors and this variability is often taken into account through the measurement of plasma concentrations in patients for individualization of dosage.

4.1 Individual pharmacokinetics

Human body represents an open dynamic system with many underlying time and substance dependent processes. Several factors like *age*, *weight* and *sex* of the subject affect this system. Size of tissue, volume of tissue fluids, perfusion of various tissues including the organs of elimination (which in turn is influenced by changes in cardiac output), the functional capacity of liver and permeability of tissue membranes also contribute in affecting the pharmacokinetics of drugs.

Many drugs (e.g. antibiotics, digoxin) are more slowly eliminated in newborns than in adults because the functional capacity of the elimination organs is not fully reached. Biotransformation which is genetically determined exhibits variation among different individuals. For example the metabolism of isoniazid, hydralazine, procainamide and some sulfonamides is either rapid or slow depending on the phenotype. It has been found that certain oxidative metabolic pathways (e.g. metabolism of sparteine/debrisoquine, mephenytoin) are also genetically determined and certain subpopulations (5–8%) can be characterized as poor or deficient metabolisers (PMs), whereas the rest are efficient metabolisers (EMs).

The environmental factors, including food habits and nutritional status as well as physical exercise can influence drug action.

Similarly, it may be expected that circadian rhythms in hormonal concentration changes and pharmacokinetics could also be of some significance.

Disease is another important factor which can influence the pharmacokinetics and -dynamics of drugs. Even though most of pharmacokinetic data available in literature are from studies conducted in healthy subjects the importance of influence of disease states like cardiac insufficiency, kidney or liver dysfunction has been well recognized and recently more investigations are made in this direction.

All these factors which may possibly influence the drug effect, make the predictions of intensity and duration of action for a given dose very difficult. The most disturbing factors that affect dose–effect relationship appear to be the individual pharmacokinetics with all above stated variations and imbalances. This problem is more alarming in case of certain drugs with a narrow therapeutic index and it is considered important to monitor plasma concentrations and to correspondingly adjust the dosage regimen in therapy involving them.

4.2 Population kinetics

It is too expensive to monitor plasma levels and to describe pharmacokinetics in every individual patient. Efforts have been made during the last few years to develop methods to derive the most important parameters in well defined patient populations. One such procedure that has been developed by Sheiner and his co-workers makes use of the information from the routinely estimated plasma concentrations. Different pharmacokinetic parameters in a population are computed based on this data using various mathematical and statistical methods. A dosage prediction is then made taking these parameters into consideration. Such data have been made available for some drugs (e.g. digoxin, phenytoin, mexilitine, theophylline, gentamicin) which are supplementary to the studies conducted in healthy subjects.

4.3 Therapeutic plasma level monitoring

Every drug therapy should be controlled in some way. The physician assesses the efficacy of the chosen therapy based on either clinical findings or laboratory estimations and correspondingly adjusts the dosage regimen for optimum response. For some drugs such an assessment is not possible as their pharmacological response cannot be exactly measured. It is potentially dangerous to alter the dosage of some drugs with narrow therapeutic range based on empirical observations as it may lead to either toxic effects or ineffective treatment. In such difficult situations measurement of plasma concentrations during therapy is desirable. It is observed that many drugs produce therapeutic effects in a certain concentration range and toxic effects beyond that. The so called "therapeutic range" for different drugs has been determined (Table 16) taking the ineffective as well as toxic levels into consideration.

The intensity of drug action is dependent on how high the plasma concentrations reach within the therapeutic range (Fig. 14). By taking the measured

Table 16. Therapeutic range of some drugs which have a narrow therapeutic index

Drug	Therapeutic concentrations	
Aprindine	1–2	mg/L
Carbamazepin	3–10	mg/L
Cyclosporine	0.1–0.4	mg/L
Digoxin	0.7–2	μg/L
Digitoxin	10–30	μg/L
Disopyramide	2–5	mg/L
Ethosuximide	50–80	mg/L
Lidocaine	1.5–4.5	mg/L
Lithium	0.5–1.1	mval/L
Mexilitine	0.8–2	mg/L
Methotrexate	5	μmol/L (24 h);
	0.9	μmol/L (48 h)
Phenytoin	7–20	mg/L
Procainamide	3.5–9	mg/L
Phenobarbital	10–30	mg/L
Primidone (+Phenobarbital)	4–10	mg/L
Quinidine	2–5	mg/L
Salicylate	20–100	mg/L (analgesic & antipyretic)
	100–250	mg/L (antiinflammatory)
Theophylline	8–20	mg/L
Tocainide	6–15	mg/L
Valproic acid	50–100	mg/L

In case of aminoglycosides the following values should not be exceeded:

	C_{min} (trough)	and	C_{max} (peak)
Amikacin	<4 mg/L		20–30 mg/L
Gentamicin	<2 mg/L		5–10 mg/L
Netilmicin	<2 mg/L		5–10 mg/L
Sisomicin	<2 mg/L		5–10 mg/L
Tobramycin	<2 mg/L		5–10 mg/L
Vancomycin	<15 mg/L		25–40 mg/L

plasma levels into consideration the variability in individual pharmacokinetics is eliminated and the intensity of action is better predictable (Fig. 15).

This approach has made the handling of drugs especially with narrow therapeutic range, which sometimes exhibit pharmacokinetic peculiarities safer and more effective (see Table 17). Following are some general indications which serve as guidelines to decide whether it is necessary to measure plasma levels or not for the optimization of dosage.

(1) Insufficient therapeutic effect, which is possibly due to insufficient dose and/or non-compliance on the part of patient and/or incomplete absorption.
(Question: Is the drug reaching plasma at all? or Is the patient not responding to treatment?)

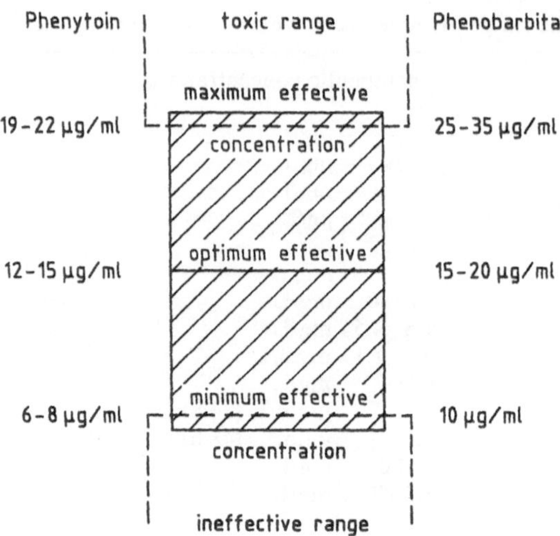

Fig. 14. The so called "therapeutic window" (of e.g. phenytoin, phenobarbital). The therapeutic range with its floating and overlapping boundaries lies between ineffective (below) and toxic (above) levels

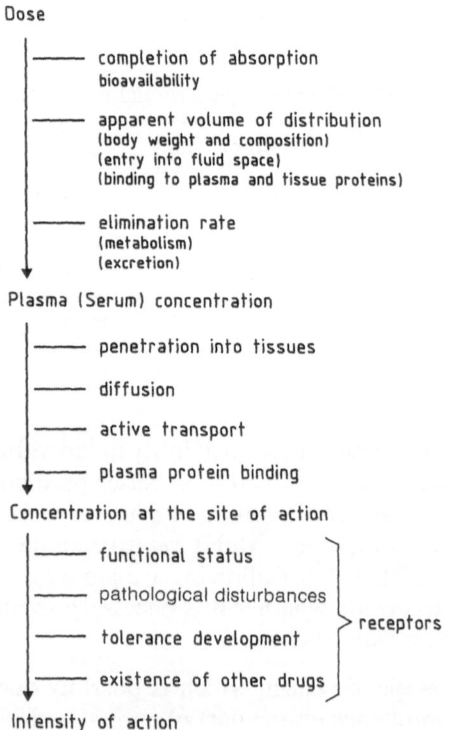

Fig. 15. The relationship between dose and intensity of action with the factors, which influence it. By measuring the plasma/serum concentrations of the drug, the variability in individual pharmacokinetics can be eliminated

(2) On suspicion of an attempt of suicide or poisoning.
(Question: Which drug has been consumed?)

(3) Dosage monitoring in diseases (renal or hepatic disorder), which may lead to accumulation of drug in body.
(Question: Whether the expected concentrations are reached or Are the concentrations abnormally high?)

(4) Dosage monitoring in case of drugs with narrow margin of safety.
(Question: same as under 3).

(5) Differential diagnosis of disease symptoms and toxic side effects due to overdosage.
(Question: Are the concentrations of drug in plasma too high?)

The measurement of plasma concentrations is unnecessary, when the therapeutic response is satisfactory or when the drug has been ingested just before plasma sampling (Table 17).

Therapeutic plasma level measurements are not "screening methods" and drug action is not simply a linear function of concentration (see page 89). Therefore a change in steady state concentration need not necessarily bring about a proportional change in pharmacological effect and it is not always possible to correlate the pharmacodynamic effect and plasma concentrations (e.g. antihypertensive effect of diazoxide, inhibition of thrombocyte aggregation by salicylate). In addition, the situation can be complicated by many factors such as considerable delay in reaching equilibrium between concentrations in plasma and at the site of action, formation of active metabolite(s), tolerance and hysteresis phenomenon (see page 90). The following suggestions will be helpful in the interpretation of results.

(1) The "therapeutic range" is an arbitrary range based on controlled trials and experience. It is a statistical range which in most patients corresponds to desired effect of drug, without appearance of dangerous side effects or toxicity. Values under this range may not be ineffective and the values above need not be toxic in each case.

(2) The "therapeutic range" need not be the same in all patients. Disease, change in electrolyte concentrations, and other factors can influence drug

Table 17. Which drugs should be measured in plasma for treatment control?

a) With narrow therapeutic range	E. g. Digitalis, Theophylline, Anticonvulsants, Antiarrhythmics, Lithium, Aminoglycosides, Cytostatics
b) Non-linear pharmacokinetics	E.g. Phenytoin, Carbamazepin
c) Inhibitors or inducers of microsomal enzymes	E.g. Dipropylacetate, Phenobarbital
d) Over or under dosing to ascertain reasons for side effects/ineffectiveness	

action. For example, the toxic effects of digoxin appear even in lower concentrations when there is simultaneous hypokalaemia or hypercalcaemia.

(3) Mostly, the estimated therapeutic range is based on the total plasma concentrations. In case of drugs which are bound to proteins, it is the unbound fraction which is pharmacologically effective. Reduced protein binding (total concentrations being still in therapeutic range) can often lead to toxic effects. This can happen in renal or hepatic diseases and in presence of displacing drugs. Phenytoin is a typical example, which has a lower therapeutic range for total drug levels in patients with renal failure.

(4) The therapeutic range is related only to measured concentrations of parent drug and it does not take the concentrations of pharmacologically active metabolite (e.g. phenobarbital in therapy with primidone, N-acetylprocainamide in case of procainamide) into consideration. These active metabolites can for example in renal failure reach higher concentrations and produce toxic effects (even though the parent drug concentrations are in normal range).
(13 to 40 nM/l). Factors which enhance the individual myocardial sensitivity to

Based on these grounds it is important that the pharmacokinetic properties of such drugs are to be carefully examined before starting the therapy. Important pharmacokinetic data of drugs for which the routine therapeutic plasma level monitoring is undertaken are summarized as follows.

Digitalis glycosides: Digoxin (about 25%) and digitoxin (about 90%) are bound to plasma proteins. The plasma half-life of digoxin is between 1.5 to 2 days and that of digitoxin is about 5 to 7 days. Digoxin about 2/3 and digitoxin about 1/3 (of administered dose) are excreted unchanged in urine. Digitoxin undergoes enterohepatic circulation and a small portion (about 5%) is biotransformed to digoxin in liver. The therapeutic range for digoxin lies between 0.7 to 2.0 ng/ml (0.9 to 2.6 nM/l) and for digitoxin between 10 to 30 ng/ml (13 to 40 nM/l). Factors which enhance the individual myocardial sensitivity to digitalis glycosides are hypokalemia, hypercalcemia, hypomagnesemia, myocardial disease, hypoxia and alkalosis. Newborn and infants show a greater tolerance to digitalis glycosides, therefore the therapeutic range in this age group is about 20% higher than in adults.

Quinidine: About 80% of administered dose is metabolised and the rest is excreted unchanged in urine depending upon urinary pH. The rate of metabolism in liver shows a wide intraindividual variation which contributes to the variation in elimination rate. Protein binding is between 70 to 80% and the normal half-life is about 6 h. The therapeutic range of quinidine lies between 2 to 5 µg/mL (6 to 15 µM/L), and dosage should be adjudged also on the clinical picture (including ECG).

Lidocaine: In plasma about 50% is bound to proteins and normally it is metabolised to monoethylglycinexylidide (MEGX) in liver with a half-life of about 100 min. The renal elimination of unchanged form is ($<2\%$) negligible.

The clearance of lidocaine under conditions of reduced hepatic perfusion (e.g. congestive heart failure, liver cirrhosis, shock) is severely impaired. MEGX is nearly as active as the parent compound but also neurotoxic and it is ultimately converted into inactive glycinexylidide. Therefore, in patients with cardiac insufficiency accumulation of MEGX can take place leading to severe toxic effects (though lidocaine concentrations are apparently in normal range). The therapeutic range of lidocaine lies between 1.5 to 4.5 μg/ml (6 to 20 μM/L). In higher concentrations there is an increased risk of toxic effects (e.g. vertigo, drowsiness, tinnitis, muscular irritability, convulsions and respiratory depression).

Procainamide: In some countries procainamide is seldom used particularly because of the great influence of variations in renal and hepatic function on its kinetics. Its metabolism shows genetic variations (acetylator phenotype). About 15% is bound to the plasma proteins and it is metabolised in liver into active N-acetylprocainamide (NAPA). The plasma half-life is about 3 to 5 h. Pharmacologically NAPA (about 10 to 15% is bound to proteins) is equally effective and it is essentially eliminated through kidneys with a half-life of 6 to 11 h. As the $t_{1/2}$ is relatively longer it poses the problem of accumulation. Therefore, chronic administration of procainamide in patients with renal failure can be potentially hazardous. For this reason, measurement of plasma levels of procainamide alone does not suffice and the levels of NAPA should also be simultaneously measured (at least in patients with renal failure). The therapeutic concentrations of procainamide lie between 3.5 to 9 μg/mL (15 to 40 μM/L) and those of NAPA have not been exactly defined. Adverse effects are, however, not so commonly observed as long as the sum of concentrations of procainamide and NAPA at any time does not exceed 30 μg/mL.

Methotrexate: Following intravenous administration elimination of methotrexate (MTX) takes place in three phases. A rapid distribution phase (with $t_{1/2}$ of about 1 h), is followed by a concentration dependent slower elimination phase. The half-life during the phase-2 is about 3 to 5 h and the terminal half-life (phase-3) is about 27 to 70 h. Longer terminal half-life is probably due to enterohepatic circulation of MTX and/or its metabolites or binding of MTX to dihydrofolate reductase. 90% of administered dose is excreted unchanged in urine. Mostly the slower elimination rather than the total dose is accountable for the toxic effects of MTX. Therefore, therapy with MTX has to be very carefully supervised and the plasma concentrations are to be monitored under the following conditions:

(1) In therapy with high doses of MTX: to supervise plasma concentration profile for 24 to 48 h following administration.
(2) In MTX intoxication: to supervise the plasma levels for 72 h or even later after administration together with leucovorin rescue procedures:

- a 24 h level below 5×10^{-6} M (<5 μM/L)
- a 48 h level below 9×10^{-7} M (<0.9 μM/L)

In general these upper levels do not result in toxic effects. If the 48 h concentration is above 9×10^{-7} M, then the rescue procedures should be immediately undertaken by simultaneously measuring MTX plasma levels or until the 72 h level falls below 3×10^{-7} M (0.3 μM/L).

Theophylline: In adults about 60% is bound to plasma proteins. Cirrhotics and premature babies show a reduced binding capacity. Elimination takes place predominantly by hepatic metabolism. Plasma half-life of theophylline in non-smokers is about 3 to 6 h and it is very much prolonged in premature babies and patients with congestive heart failure. The systemic clearance shows fluctuations because of various influences. In addition, co-administration of drugs like erythromycin, oleandomycin, cimetidine, thiabendazole, oral contraceptives, β-blockers and allopurinol reduce the clearance by inhibiting the metabolism. Rifampicin, carbamazepin, phenytoin and barbiturates on the other hand, increase the clearance by inducing the metabolism. The therapeutic range lies between 8 to 20 μg/mL (45 to 110 μM/L) for adults and children, however, in premature babies because of low protein binding it lies between 6 to 11 μg/mL (33 to 60 μM/L). Toxic symptoms such as nausea, headache, abdominal pain, diarrhoea, fall in B.P, restlessness and sinustachycardia appear when the concentrations are above 20 μg/mL (110 μM/L). In much higher concentrations there is a danger of tachyarrhythmia and epileptic seizures.

Anticonvulsants: The pharmacokinetic data of individual substances are given in Table 18. The elimination rates exhibit a great variation because of capacity limited elimination (e.g. phenytoin) and self induction (e.g. carbamazepine, phenobarbital; Table 18).

Salicylates: Analgesic/antipyretic and antiinflammatory effects are produced in the concentration (in terms of salicylic acid) ranges 20 to 100 μg/mL (120 to 600 μM/L) and 100 to 250 μg/mL (600 to 1500 μM/L) respectively. In concentrations above 300 μg/mL (1650 μM/L) undesirable effects such as tinnitis, nausea, hyperventilation and agitation are produced. As long as the concentrations are below 400 μg/mL (2400 μM/L) these effects can be controlled and if they reach beyond 470 μg/ml (2600 μM/L) life threatening metabolic acidosis may result. Practically all salicylates, following absorption are converted to salicyclic acid and are partly (dose dependent) biotransformed. In analgesic concentration range $t_{1/2}$ is 2 to 3 h and in higher concentrations it may reach 15 to 30 h. The renal elimination is considerably high only when the urine is alkaline (30 to 80% of dose).

Lithium: It is eliminated unchanged by renal filtration and tubular reabsorption. Excretion can be accelerated by an increased Na^+ uptake. The unbound fraction of lithium is rapidly and completely reabsorbed and it is eliminated with a half-life of 22 h (10 to 35 h depending on the renal function). The steady state concentrations are reached in 4 to 5 days. For therapeutic effect the

Table 18. Pharmacokinetic characterization of some anticonvulsants

	Carbamazepine	Phenytoin [a]	Phenobarbital	Primidone [b]	Valproic acid	Ethosuximide
Therap. range						
mg/L	3–10	7–20	10–30	4–10	50–100	50–80
μmol/L	13–42	28–80	45–130	18–46	345–710	350–570
Time to reach steady state [c]	1–2 w	1–3 w	2–3 w	0.5 w	0.5 w	1–2 w
Protein binding (%)	75	90	50	20	90	5
Renal elimination [d] (%)	0	0	20	0	0	20
Half-life (h)	12–24	12–40	60–120	10–12	10–20	30–60

w, weeks
[a] Phenytoin exhibits non-linear kinetics, therefore in higher doses the elimination half life depends upon the plasma concentrations.
[b] Active metabolites of primidone are phenobarbital and PEMA! Therefore it is required to measure at least additionally phenobarbital in plasma.
[c] All epileptics other than valproic acid and ethosuximide induce hepatic drug metabolism.
[d] Excreted unchanged in urine (% of dose).

plamsa concentration measured 12 ± 1 h after should be between 0.5 to 0.8 m val/L. Concentrations above 1.5 m val/L may produce severe side effects.

Cyclosporine A: Pharmacokinetics of cyclosporine A exhibit great interindividual variation. The drug may be measured in plasma, serum or blood by different methods including radio immuno assay (RIA) and high performance liquid chromatography (HPLC) with variable specificity. Following oral administration it is slowly (t_{max} is about 3.5 h) and incompletely absorbed (12 to 35%). Cyclosporine is strongly bound to plasma proteins (about 80%) and the blood-plasma concentration ratio is nearly 2. It is metabolised by hydroxylation and N-demethylation in liver with a blood clearance of 5 to 13 mL/min/kg. The terminal half-life is about 6 to 25 h and it is excreted in bile. For this drug it is very difficult to define an exact therapeutic range, which depends upon the method used for the determination of concentrations and the nature of biological material (serum/blood). However, the optimum blood concentrations lie between 100 to 300 μg/mL (HPLC method) and serum concentrations lie between 100 to 400 μg/mL (RIA method).

Aminoglycosides: Gentamicin, netilmicin, tobramicin and amikacin have nephro- and ototoxic properties. The therapeutic and toxic concentrations lie very close to each other. The normal $t_{1/2}$ is between 1.5 to 3 h. They are essentially eliminated unchanged in urine, therefore their clearance is nearly proportional to creatinine clearance. The nephrotoxicity of these drugs is due to accumulation in deeper compartments (e.g. kidneys). Peak plasma concentrations (C_{max}) depending on the dose administered are reached in about 1 h following i.m. administration. C_{min} (the concentration before the administration of next dose) is dependent on dosing interval and renal function. The peak concentrations in the range of 5 to 10 μg/mL (10 to 20 μM/L) are considered effective. C_{min} should be below 2 μg/mL, so that no undesired effects are produced. In case of amikacin the therapeutic range lies between 20 to 25 μg/mL (34 to 43 μM/L) and C_{min} should be below 4 μg/mL (7 μM/L).

4.4 Individual dose determination

Dettli developed a method of estimation the individual elimination rate, which helps in optimization of dosage of drugs which are essentially eliminated by kidneys (e.g. digoxin, antibiotics). The mathematical relationship is given as (also see page 43)

$$CL_{ind} = CL_H + \alpha' \cdot CL_{cr} \tag{115}$$

where

CL_{ind} = individual clearance
CL_H = hepatic clearance (population mean)
CL_{cr} = individual creatinine clearance
α' = proportionality factor derived from a kinetic study, if possible conducted in patients with varying renal function

Based on the above expression a dosage regimen for gentamicin was developed, but it was not precise enough because of very high interindividual variability in elimination even in subjects with normal renal function. Similarly the dosage regimen of digoxin was also investigated in individual subjects by using different nomograms. Many other studies conducted in similar way, however, showed that the predictions made using nomograms based on serum creatinine, sex, age, body weight and height resulted in inaccurate dosage because of very large interindividual variability in V (about 35%) and CL (about 50%).

A nomogram based on population data, for theophylline was developed, which could also not give accurate predictions because of various factors (e.g. nutrition, smoking, acute diseases, drugs) that influence the individual elimination. Therefore, there is a need for a suitable method, which enables prediction of a dosage regimen that produces C_{av}^{ss} in therapeutic range, with minimum fluctuations. Some of the available methods are discussed here.

In the simplest case, the dose is altered based on the relation between the desired and the measured plasma levels (in steady state the average concentration is porportional to the maintenance dose; $C_{av}^{ss} \sim DM$, provided CL remains constant). This method, however, is applicable only when the measured concentration lies between 70 and 150% of the desired level.

A better approach involves pharmacokinetic investigation following i.v. administration of a test dose. This approach has been successfully applied for drugs like methotrexate, theophylline and tobramycin. The variation between the desired and actually measured C_{av}^{ss} has been found to be around 20–25%.

A more simple approach based on empirical observations or studies involves only one measured plasma concentration. This was applied to drugs like lithium, impiramine and desmethylimpiramine. The plasma concentration measured within 24 h of initial dose administration and C_{av}^{ss} have shown a significant correlation (the variability is only about 15%). Similarly the variation has been found to be very low (around 20%) between simulated C^{ss} and actually measured values (from literature) in patients treated with theophylline and chloramphenicol. For aminoglycosides, the information obtained from general patient data was combined with plasma concentration measurements to make a dosage prediction by this method. However, it has been observed that for more exact predictions at least 3 measurements are necessary.

The population parameters obtained from routine data can be used along with the actually measured plasma levels for optimization of individual dosage ("Bayesian approach"). To achieve this, the mean values of population kinetic parameters with their variability must be available. It is then possible to calculate the theoretically expected concentrations (see Fig. 16). By comparing the expected and actually measured levels the kinetic parameters (subsequently used for dosage predictions) in individual patients can be assessed. If the actually measured concentration deviates very much from the expected one, the reasons (e.g. irregular or inappropriate dosing) for such a discrepancy should be investigated. Besides kinetic reasons, the plasma sampling and the method of drug estimation may also sometimes contribute to the variations. Phenytoin and digoxin were employed as model drugs for comparison of

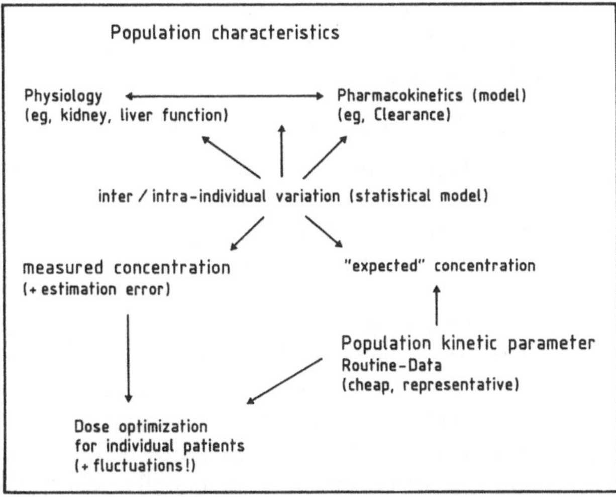

Fig. 16. The interrelationship between physiology, pharmacokinetics, population-kinetic data and monitored plasma concentrations, which lead to the individual dose optimization

Bayesian method with the others. This approach has also been applied recently to a relatively new antiarrhythmic drug, mexiletine. The variability in this case has been found to be 20 to 30%.

These modern methods are based on simplified and linearized statistical and pharmacokinetic assumptions. As these studies are usually conducted in a small number of patients generalization of results is difficult, because the data of an individual patient may deviate from the assumed model; all methods can provide only a "best fit" to the clinical, highly variable releality.

4.5 Effect kinetics

More recently relationships between onset, duration and intensity of drug action and changes in plasma concentrations have received increasing attention (often referred to as "effect kinetics"). Many peculiarities are observed in the concentration–effect relationship and they are to be properly interpreted from actual data obtained.

Following linear models, the pharmacodynamic response (E_{dyn}) is directly proportional to the concentration in plasma C

$$E_{dyn} = S \cdot C \qquad (116)$$

where S represents the slope of the regression line.

This method does not define a "maximal effect" and the relationship between concentration–effect is meaningful only within the measured range.

In another model, the so called "E_{max}-model" a maximal effect (E_{max}) is predicted and there is no effect at concentration zero.

$$E_{dyn} = E_{max} \cdot C/(EC_{50} + C) \qquad (117)$$

where EC_{50} is the concentration corresponding to 50% of maximal effect.

A variation of this model represents the so called "sigmoidal E_{max}-model", which can be expressed as follows

$$E_{dyn} = E_{max} \cdot C^N/(EC_{50}^N + C^N) \qquad (118)$$

where the exponent N is Hill coefficient which influences the slope and the form of concentration–effect curve. The above equation is known as Hill's equation.

This model is more advantageous than the others for describing the pharmacological effects and it also enables interpretation in the effect range of 20 to 80%.

Some examples which have clinical relevance are illustrated as follows.

In case of d-tubocurarine concentration–effect curve, three phases can be observed (see Fig. 17). During the first phase (region 3) it can be seen that there is a sustained maximal effect even though the concentration is falling exponentially. During the second phase the effect goes down linearly with time and during the third (region 1) both concentration as well as effect fall exponentially. It is actually in the third phase that one finds a direct proportionality between concentration and effect (Fig. 17).

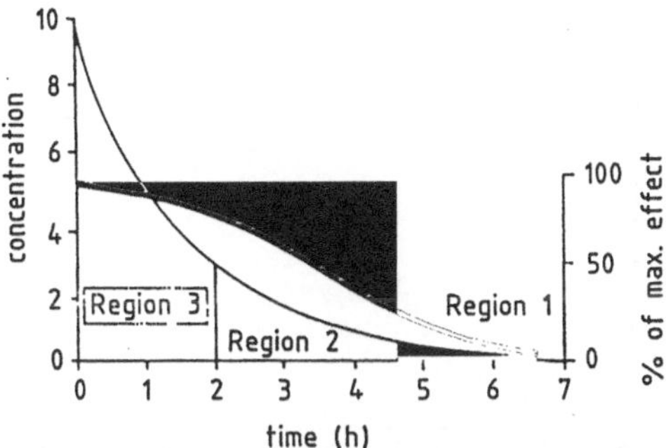

Fig. 17. The relationship between drug concentration (thin line) and pharmacological effect (thick line) after i.v. administration of tubocurarine (modified after Rowland et al., 1980)

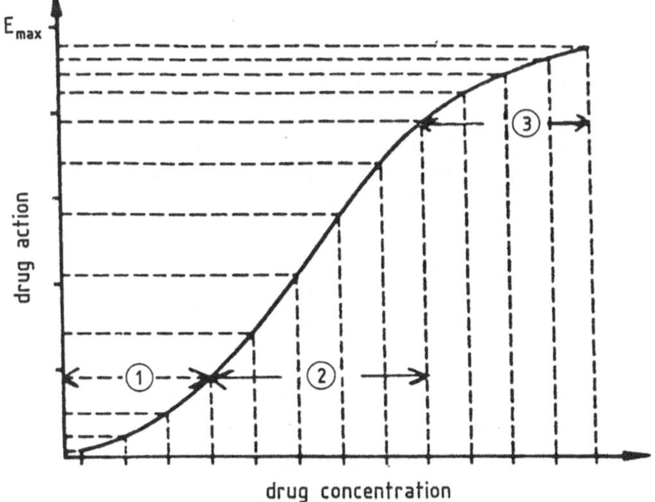

Fig. 18. Typical relationship between the intensity of action and the plasma concentration of a drug, with three characteristic regions. The change in intensity with increase in concentration is more remarkable at the middle region than at the lower and the upper regions

Usually the classical dose-response curve is represented semilogarithmically as shown in Fig. 18, where again three phases can be differentiated. The dose–effect relationship appears to be nearly linear intitially and becomes exponential during the later phase (which amounts to 20 to 80%) of maximal effect. During the last phase the increase in effect with dose is very small. The concentration–effect curves in the entire range can be generated with the help of computer programs, using the Hill's equation.

Another possibility of representing effect relationships is by "all or none" approach. Figure 19 shows the dose-response curve of propranolol in patients with ventricular arrhythmias, where the ordinate represents frequency of ther-

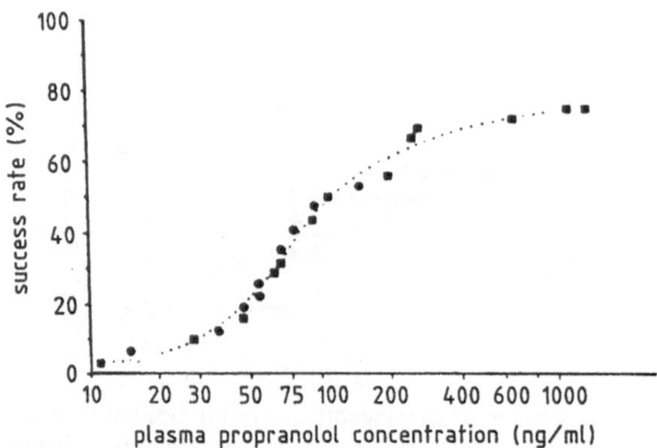

Fig. 19. Concentration–effect relationship between propranolol plasma concentration and antiarrhythmic effect (expressed as % success rate) investigated in outpatients (●) and stationary patients (■), receiving a daily dose between 80 and 640 mg/die (after Woosely et al., 1979)

apeutic success expressed as percentage. The therapeutic effect shows an increase up to 70% suppression of arrhythmias with increasing dose of drug. The maximum administered daily dose was 940 mg. The curve shows that 70% of the patients responded to the treatment and in about 40% of the patients suppression of arrhythmias occurred at concentrations above 100 ng/mL. The fact that β-blockade is already maximal at 100 ng/mL shows that suppression of ventricular arrhythmias takes place through some other mechanism. Further invasive electrophysiological investigations revealed that at concentrations beyond 100 ng/mL an increasing "membrane stabilising effect" is produced.

Deviations in the classical form of dose-response curve are mainly found immediately following the administration of a drug. It is often observed that the drug effect shows an increase when the plasma concentrations actually start

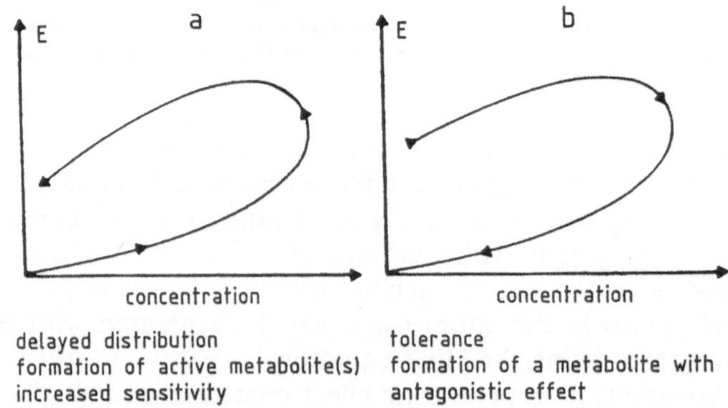

Fig. 20 a, b. Concentration–effect relationships in the form of hysteresis loops (anticlockwise and clock-wise)

declining. This is due to the fact that the equilibrium between plasma and receptor sites is delayed with respect to the administered drug. In such cases the effect–concentration curve exhibits the shape of a hysteresis loop (anti-clockwise) when related to time (see Fig. 20a). An anticlockwise hysteresis loop can imply delayed distribution or slow formation of an active metabolite (e.g. isosorbide mononitrate from isosorbide dinitrate) or increased sensitivity of receptors (e.g. long term infusion of lower dose of angiotensin). On the other hand, a clockwise hysteresis loop can mean that there is an accumulation of an antagonist or development of tolerance by the receptors to the drug (see Fig. 20b).

In case of metoprolol, the decrease in heart rate corresponding to a particular concentration following administration of 100 mg is less remarkable than that corresponding to the same concentration following administration of 50 mg. It may be speculated that the accumulation of a metabolite with antagonistic effect is more pronounced after the larger dose.

Concentration–effect curves may be also influenced by route of administration of drug. In case of lorcainide, the concentration response curve following p.o. administration shows a greater shift towards left than following i.v. administration suggesting the formation of an active metabolite due to first pass effect. If the formation of an active metabolite is rate limiting, the effect produced will be parallel to the kinetics of the parent substance. In such an instance it may be wrongly concluded that the parent substance is active. The fact that the metabolite is effective can be demonstrated when the concentration–effect curve shows a significant shift towards left following its direct administration if compared to the parent substance.

Inverse effects are observed in case of verapamil. A more significant prolongation of PQ interval in ECG is noticed following i.v. administration than following p.o. administration. It may be explained that racemic verapamil undergoes a stereoselective first pass effect. The more effective L-form, is metabolised faster than the less effective D-form. This results in a D/L ratio of 2 following i.v. administration and 5 following p.o. administration. Thus, following i.v. administration the more potent L-form is available in relatively higher concentrations.

If there is no correlation between concentration and effect it should be ascertained whether the measured parameter represents primary pharmacological effect of the drug or whether the effect is produced through some indirect mechanism. The specific examples should indicate that essential information about a drug can be obtained only if its pharmacokinetics will be also related to effect. The deviations in the dose-response curve from the classical form can be often explained if the above discussed factors are taken into consideration.

Part III

Appendix

1 Recommended pharmacokinetic symbols, definitions and dimensions

New standard symbol	Definition and dimension	Other symbols
A	Amount of drug in the body at any given time t (mass).	A
A^{ss}	Amount of drug in the body at steady state (mass).	A_{ss}
Ae	Amount of unchanged drug excreted into urine (mass).	A_e, A_u, D_u
Ae(∞)	Amount of unchanged drug excreted into urine upto time infinity (mass).	Ae, D_u, X_u
AUC	Area under the plasma concentration – time curve from zero to infinity (mass · time/volume).	$AUC_{0\to\infty}$
AUC(0–t)	Area under the concentration – time curve from zero to time t (mass · time/volume).	$AUC_{0\to t}$
AUC_{τ}^{ss}	Area under the concentration – time curve in steady state during a dosing interval (mass · time/volume).	$AUC_{0-\tau}$
C	Drug concentration in plasma (mass/volume).	c, c_p, c_t, Y
C_1	Ordinate intercept of the residual line (from the differences between the concentrations during the most rapid initial phase and the extrapolated later phase) (mass/volume).	A, A_1, C_2
C_z	Ordinate intercept of the terminal elimination line (mass/volume).	B, A_2, C_1
C(0)	Initial (fictitious) plasma concentration following a rapid i.v. injection (mass/volume).	c_0, Y^0
C_{max}	Maximum (peak) plasma concentration after single dose administration (mass/volume).	c_{max}, c_pK
$C_{max(N)}$	Maximum (peak) plasma concentration after a given number of doses (N) before steady state is reached (mass/volume).	$c_{max\,N}$, $Y_{max\,N}$
$C_{min(N)}$	Minimum (trough) plasma concentration after repetitive dosing (N) before steady state is reached (mass/volume).	$c_{min\,N}$, $Y_{min\,N}$
C(t)	Plasma concentration at any time t (mass/volume).	c_t
C^{ss}	Steady state concentration in plasma during constant rate infusion (mass/volume).	C_{ss}, C_{SS}
C_{av}^{ss}	Mean or average steady state concentration in plasma during multiple dosing (mass/volume).	c, c_{SS}, c_{pSS}

(Continued)

New standard symbols	Definition and dimension	Other symbols
C^{ss}_{max}	Peak steady state drug concentration in plasma during multiple dosing (mass/volume).	c'_{max}, C_{max}
C^{ss}_{min}	Minimum (trough) steady state drug concentration plasma during multiple dosing (mass/volume).	c'_{min}, C_{min}
CL	Total body clearance of drug from plasma (volume/time) or (volume/time / body weight).	Cl_t, C^1, TBC, Vpl, CL_B
CL_H	Hepatic clearance of drug from plasma (volume/time).	Cl_H, Cl_{hep}
CL_{int}	Intrinsic hepatic clearance of free (unbound) drug in plasma (volume/time).	Cl_{int}, $Cl_{hep.int}$
CL_{NR}	Non-renal clearance of drug from plasma (volume/time).	Cl_{nonren}, $Cl_{extraren}$
CL_R	Renal clearance from plasma (volume/time).	Cl_{ren}, Cl^R, V_{CLr}
CL_{CR}	Creatinine clearance (volume/time).	Cl_{cr}, Cr_{cl}, CIC Cl_{creat}
D	Dose size (mass).	D, Dose
DL	Loading dose (mass).	D_L, D*
DM	Maintenance dose (mass).	D_M, D_m, D
E	Organ extraction ratio.	E
F	Fraction of administered dose systemically available (or bioavailability).	f, FF*
f_a	Fraction of administered dose absorbed.	f, F′
f_e	Fraction of unchanged drug excreted in urine.	F_{el}, f, F
f_{fp}	Fraction of the absorbed dose which reached systemic circulation after first-pass effect.	f_{FPE}, F*
f_m	Fraction of drug metabolised.	f_{met}, F_{met}
f_u	Free (unbound) fraction of drug in plasma.	F, f, F_{free}
k	First order rate constant ($time^{-1}$).	k_1, k′, Kr
k_a	Absorption rate constant ($time^{-1}$).	ka, K_a, k_{01}
k_m	Rate constant (first order) for formation of metabolite ($time^{-1}$).	k_{met}, K_M
Km	Michaelis-Menten constant (mass/volume).	k_m, K_m
k_e	Rate constant (first order) for unchanged drug appearing in urine ($time^{-1}$).	k_u, k_{el}
k_0	Zero order rate constant (mass/volume).	k^0, K_0
k_{10}	Elimination rate constant (first order) from central (1) compartment ($time^{-1}$).	k_{el}, k_e, k_{13}, k_d, K_2
k_{12}	Transfer rate constant from the central (1) to peripheral (2) compartment ($time^{-1}$).	k_1, K_{12}

(Continued)

New standard symbols	Definition and dimension	Other symbols
k_{21}	Transfer rate constant from the peripheral (2) to central (1) compartment ($time^{-1}$).	k_2, K_{21}
λ_1	Largest disposition (hybrid) rate constant ($time^{-1}$).	α, λ_2, γ_1
λ_z	Smallest disposition (hybrid) rate constant ($time^{-1}$).	β, λ_1, γ_2
Q_H	Liver blood flow (volume/time).	Q, Q_{hep}, LBF
Q_R	Renal blood flow (volume/time).	RBF
R_0	Constant infusion rate (mass/time).	K^0, k^0, R^0
t	Time after drug administration (time).	T
t_{lag}	Lag-time (time).	T_{lag}, T2
t_{max}	Time to reach peak (maximum) concentration following drug administration (time).	t_p, T_{max}
$t_{1/2a}$	Absorption half-life (time).	t_a, $t_{1/2}$
$t_{1/2\,\lambda_i}$	Half-life corresponding to the ith phase of a polyexponential function (time).	$T_{1/2a}$, $t_{1/2}$
$t_{1/2}$	Elimination half-life associated with the terminal slope of a semi-log concentration-time curve ($time^{-1}$).	$T_{1/2}$, $T_{50\%}$, $t_{1/2\beta}$, $T_{1/2\beta}$
τ	Dosing interval (time).	
V_c	Pharmacokinetic volume of central compartment (volume).	V_p, V_1, V
V_z	Volume of distribution during terminal phase (volume).	V_d, Vd_β, Vd_{area}
V_{ss}	Volume of distribution at steady state (volume).	Vd_{SS}, V_{SS}
V_{max}	Maximum rate of metabolism by an enzyme mediated reaction (concentration/time).	Vm

Symbol Qualifiers

Sites of Measurement
(to qualify C, CL, AUC, etc.):

p	plasma
b	blood
u	unbound species
sal	saliva
ur	urine
t	tissue

Organs and elimination routes
(to qualify CL, k, Q, *f*, etc):

H	hepatic
R	renal
NR	non-renal
e	excreted into urine
m	metabolised

Routes of administration
(to qualify D, DL, DM, AUC, etc.):

iv	intravenous
po	peroral
sc	subcutaneous
im	intramuscular
sl	sublingual
rect	rectal
ip	intraperitoneal

2 Glossary

Absolute bioavailability is the fraction of the dose of a drug substance in a dosage form absorbed into the systemic circulation following extravascular administration when the reference is the same dose of drug administered by intravenous route.

Absorption is the process of drug transfer into blood circulation across the biological membrane by active process or passive diffusion.

Accumulation is the increase in concentration of a drug in blood, plasma, serum, tissue, or the amount of drug in the body until steady state is reached.

Area Under the Curve is the area under the plasma concentration-time curve (time 0 to infinite) following administration of a single dose or the area under the curve during a dosing interval at steady state.

Bioavailability is defined as the rate at which the drug appears in the systemic circulation and the relative amount of administered dose which reaches systemic circulation.

Bioequivalence: When the rate and extent of absorption (bioavailability) of a drug from two different formulations, following administration of equimolar doses does not substantially differ the two dosage forms are said to be *bioequivalent.*

Blood flow is the rate at which blood passes through an organ or tissue (blood perfusion).

Central compartment represents the sum of all body organs and tissues in which the drug concentration approaches immediately equilibrium with that in blood, plasma or serum.

Chronopharmacokinetics is the study of the influence of circadian rhythms (controlled by endogenous factors) or disturbances in daily routine (due to external factors) on the pharmacokinetic parameters.

Clearance describes the elimination of a drug from the body. Under steady state conditions clearance is a proportionality constant relating the available dose-rate to the steady state concentration of drug in a specified body fluid (blood, plasma etc.) and elimination organ (e.g. liver, kidney).

Compartment is a hypothetical homogenous entity which can be mathematically described by a volume and its drug concentration.

Creatinine clearance is the ratio of excretion rate of creatinine in urine to the serum creatinine concentration. It is used as a measure of renal function.

Disposition includes all processes and factors which take place in the body from the time the drug reaches the circulation to the time when it, or its metabolite(s) leaves the body in urine, feces, sweat or expired air (distribution, metabolism and excretion).

Dosage regimen is the pattern of dosing (mass and interval) required to produce or/and to maintain clinical effectiveness (through therapeutic concentrations) in the body.

Dose is the amount of drug administered by any route.

Dose or concentration dependency refers to a change in one or more disposition processes with changing dose or concentration.

Dose-response curve is the graphic representation of the relationship between dose and pharmacological or toxicological effect (response).

Dosing interval is the time period between two doses.

Drug is a substance of chemical or biological origin intented for prophylactic, therapeutic or diagnostic use in human or animals.

Elimination half-life is the time required to decrease the drug concentration in blood, plasma or serum to one half by the process of elimination.

Enterohepatic recirculation refers to the cyclic process of biliary excretion of drug into intestine followed by its reabsorption into systemic circulation.

Enzyme induction is the increase in enzyme content and activity which may result in enhanced metabolism of a substance.

Enzyme inhibition is the decrease in rate of metabolism (usually competitive) of a substance by an enzyme system.

Excretion of drugs (metabolites) is the final elimination from the body into urine, feces, sweat, air, and milk, etc.

Extraction of a drug by an organ is the ratio between organ clearance and blood flow through that organ (e.g. liver, kidney).

Extravascular administration refers to all routes of administration other than those where the drug is directly introduced into the circulation. Examples of extravascular administration include intramuscular (I.M), subcutaneous (S.C), intraperitoneal (I.P), oral etc.

First-pass effect is the phenomenon of elimination (metabolism) of a part of the absorbed dose, following oral or deep rectal administration of the drug before it reaches systemic circulation.

Flip-flop model refers to the phenomenon, where the absorption rate ("input") of a drug is much smaller than the elimination rate ("output").

Generic product is a formulation of drug which is marketed with the generic name (e.g. paracetamol, acetylsalicylic acid)

Hepatic clearance is the fraction of total body clearance which is accounted for by the liver. It depends upon hepatic blood flow, unbound drug concentration in blood and intrinsic hepatic clearance.

Hybrid rate constants are composite rate constants consisting of two or more microconstants (e.g. λ_1, λ_z).

Initial dose of a drug is the dose administered at the beginning of a therapy, which is normally larger than the maintenance dose (for achieving the steady state concentration rapidly).

Intravascular administration refers to all routes where the drug is directly introduced into the systemic circulation and the bioavailability is always 100%. Examples of intravascular administrations are intravenous (i.v.), intraarterial (i.a.).

Intrinsic clearance is the theoretical maximum clearance of an unbound drug by an elimination organ, which is not restricted by perfusion of the organ.

I.V. Bolus (Push) implies a rapid intravenous administration.

Lag time is the difference between the time of drug administration and the time at which it reaches blood stream in measurable concentrations.

Lean body weight is the total body weight minus fat mass in a subject.

Loading or priming dose see initial dose.

Maintenance dose is the dose required to maintain the therapeutic concentration for a desired length time period.

Mean Residence Time (MRT) is the average duration of stay of intact drug molecules in the body. For a drug which exhibits linear kinetics MRT is expressed as the ratio between the area under the 1st statistical moment's curve (AUMC) and the area under the curve (AUC).

Michaelis-Menten Kinetics characterize certain non-linear or saturable processes usually involving enzymatic reactions.

Multiple dose administration refers to repeated administration of a drug at definite intervals of time. Accumulation may take place if the dosing interval is shorter than that required to eliminate the drug from the body.

Non-linear or saturation kinetics refer to the situation where a rate constant is not proportional to the concentration of the substrate. An example for non-linear kinetics is a capacity limited, enzyme catalyzed metabolic reaction.

Peripheral compartment represents the sum of all body regions (organs or tissues) into which a drug is distributed, but is not in immediate equilibrium with the central compartment. A peripheral compartment is also called as tissue compartment and is often subdivided into shallow and deep compartments.

Pharmacokinetics is the mathematical description of the processes that affect drug or its metabolite(s) concentrations in human or animal body.

Relative bioavailability is the relative amount of drug which reaches the systemic circulation and the relative rate at which it appears in the blood stream, when it is administered in the same subject in two or more different dosage forms following the same or different routes of administration.

Renal clearance is the fraction of the total body clearance which is accounted for by kidneys. It is determined by the net effects of glomerular filtration, tubular active secretion and reabsorption.

Steady state is a condition at which input and output of drug are equal. Strictly speaking it is achieved only during a constant intravenous infusion. During multiple dose administration the steady state concentrations fluctuate between maximum and minimum (trough) steady state concentrations within each dosing interval.

Total clearance is the sum of individual clearances of different elimination organs.

Volume of distribution is not a real volume in the body. It is a proportionality constant relating the amount or mass of drug in the body to the measured concentration in blood, plasma or serum.

3 Tables with pharmacokinetic data

The most important pharmacokinetic parameters of some drug substances[1], arranged in alphabetical order are given in the following tables. The values of different parameters mentioned in these tables, represent those of healthy adult subjects, therefore they may deviate more or less significantly from the values determined in individual patients. However, they can serve as good guide lines.

Abbreviations

$t_{1/2}$:	terminal elimination half-life
F:	bioavailability
A_e^{∞}:	amount excreted unchanged in urine
f_u:	free (unbound) fraction in plasma
CL:	total (systemic) plasma clearance
V:	apparent volume of distribution

[1] The trade names in brackets apply only in the Federal Republic of Germany.

3 Tables with pharmacokinetic data

Substance (trade name)	$t_{1/2}$ h	F %	A_e^∞ %	f_u %	CL ml/min	V l/kg	Remarks
Acebutolol (Prent, Neptal)	2.7±0.4	37±12	40±11	75	480±60	1.2±0.3	F can increase in steady state, active acetylated metabolite (diacetylol) accumulates
Acemetacin (Rantudil)	4.5±2.8			27	35±15		
Acenocoumarol (Sintrom)	10 2–4			2±0.2	21 242	0.2 0.33	R(+)Enantiomer S(−)Enantiomer
Acetazolamide (eg, Diamox)	3.5	100	90	7		0.2	
β-Acetyldigoxin (eg, Novodigal)	36–48	70–85	70	80	100–190	5–8	F of α-form 50–60%, β-form can undergo isomerisation to α-form V and CL↓ in renal insufficiency
Acetyldigitoxin	8–10 days!	70–80	50	19			
Acetylsalicylic acid (eg, Aspirin)	0.25±0.03	68±3	1.4±1.2	50	650±80	0.15±0.03	Presystemic elimination (partly) to salicylic acid
Aclaplastin	3			57			
Acyclovir (Zovirax)	2.1±0.5	15–30	62–91	85	297±53	0.57±0.08	F is dose dependent
Adriamycin (Doxorubicin)	30–45						High interindividual variation, accumulation in renal insufficiency
Alcohol	0.24±0.1	100	<3		hepatic	0.54±0.05	Non-linear kinetics with V_{max}=124±10 mg/kg/h and K_m=82±29 mg/l

Alcuronium (Alloferin)	3.3±1.3		80–85		90±26	0.3±0.1	
Alfentanil (Rapifen)	1.6±0.2		<1	10	570±180	1.0±0.3	$t_{1/2}$ ↑ in the elderly
Alprazolam (Tafil)	12		20	30	90	1.1	Delayed elimination in cirrhosis
Allopurinol (eg, Zyloric)	1.5	80	10–20	95	796±190	0.6±0.2	Active metabolite alloxanthine is eliminated by kidneys ($t_{1/2}$=17 –42 h)
Alprenolol (Aptin)	3.1±1.2	9±5	0.5	15	1100±650	3.4±1.2	F dose dependent through capacity limited first pass effect
Amantadine (eg, Symmetrel)	9–15	95	55	33		3.5	
Amfepramone (eg, Regenon)			2				Extensive first pass effect
Amikacin (eg, Biklin)	2.3±0.4		98	95	80±1.5	0.3±0.1	
Amiloride (Arumil)	9.6±1.5	50–60	100		523±96	5.2	
Aminogluthetimid (Orimeten)	12.5–19.5	75			58.1±20.7	1.04±0.37	$t_{1/2}$=7.3 h in long term treatment through enzyme induction
Aminocaproic acid (eg, Epsilon-Aminocaproic acid (Roche))	1.6±0.1	95	<5		112±9	0.22±0.03	
5-Aminosalicylic acid (see Mesalazin)							Active metabolite of salicylazo-sulfapyridine

3 Tables with pharmacokinetic data (continued)

Substance (trade name)	$t_{1/2}$ h	F %	A_e^∞ %	f_u %	CL ml/min	V 1/kg	Remarks
P.-Aminosalicylic acid (eg, PAS-Fatol)	24.4 min! i.v. 1.08 oral	90	25	85		7.4	
Amiodarone (Cordarex)	25 ± 12 days!	35–50	<1	4	8.6 ± 2	66 ± 44	$t_{1/2} = 53 \pm 24$ days as observed in patients
Amitriptyline (eg, Laroxyl)	32–40	30–70	<2	5	430 ± 120	8.3 ± 2.0	Hepatic first pass effect (30–70%) active metabolite nortriptyline ($t_{1/2} = 18–80$ h)
Amobarbital (Stadadorm)	15–30		<4	40	38–60	0.5–1.2	Active hydroxylated metabolite
Amosulalol	2.8 ± 0.1	100	25		111.5 ± 7.4	0.75 ± 0.06	
Amoxicillin (eg, Clamoxyl)	1.0 ± 0.1	93 ± 10	52 ± 15	83	380 ± 90	0.4 ± 0.2	
Amphetamine	12	100	65			4.0	
Amphotericin B (eg, Ampho-Moronal)	15 ± 2 days!		<3	<10	30 ± 6	4.0 ± 0.4	
Ampicillin (eg, Binotal)	1.3 ± 0.2	62 ± 17	80–90	82	275 ± 50	0.3 ± 0.1	$t_{1/2}$ prolonged in newborn, uremia and cirrhosis
Amrinone (Wincoram)	4.0 ± 1.6	93 ± 12	25 ± 10	60	320 ± 110	1.2 ± 0.3	
Apalcillin (Lumota)	0.7–2.0		11–26	15	138 ± 30	0.21 ± 0.04	

Aprindine (Amidonal)	13–50	90	1	10	180		
Astemizole (Hismanal)	20	100		3.3			
Atenolol (Tenormin)	6.3±1.8	56±30	85	>95	95	0.6±0.3	
Atracurium	0.35				380±70	0.15	
Atropine (eg, Atropinol)	2–4	100	50	55	530±310	2–4	
Auranofin (Ridaura)	17–25 days!	25	15	40.1	0.73		High blood–plasma ratio
Aurothioglucose (Aureothan)	5–8 days!	100		5			
Aurothiomaleate Sod. (Tauredon)	10–35 days!	100	60–90	5	490±42	0.26±0.05	
Aurothiopolypeptide (Auro-Detoxin)	27 days!	100		1.5			
Azapropazone (Prolixan)	18±5		60–70	0.5	9.2±2.5	0.2±0.1	
Azathioprine (Imurek)	0.16	60±31	<2		4000±2000	0.8±0.6	Rapid conversion to active mercaptopurine
Azidocillin (Syncillin)	0.5	75	60	17			

3 Tables with pharmacokinetic data (continued)

Substance (trade name)	$t_{1/2}$ h	F %	A_e^∞ %	f_u %	CL ml/min	V 1/kg	Remarks
Azlocillin (Securopen)	1.0±0.2		65±9	72	230±50 160±30	0.2±0.1	Following doses 30 mg/kg and 80 mg/kg respectively
Aztreonam (eg, Azactam)	1.7±0.1		66	44	108±24	0.25±0.05	
Bencyclane (Fludilat)	12			10	660	7.1	
Bendroflumethiazide (Sinesalin)	3	100	30±6	6	364±73	1.5±0.4	
Bacitracin	1.5	1	30				
Baclofen (Lioresal)	3–4	95	80	70		0.85	
Barbexaclone (Maliasin)	see Phenobarbital						Salt of phenobarbital and levopropyl hexidrine
Benoxaprofen (Coxigon)	28–48	95	4–6	0.2	Hepatic	0.14	
Benzarone (eg, Fragivex)	13.5±2.2		<1.6		Hepatic		
Benzbromarone (eg, Uricovac)	2.8±1.1	25	1		84±19	0.3±0.1	Rapid dehalogenation to active benzarone
Benzydamine (Tantum)	13	97	5	>80	169±32	1.6	

Benzylpenicillin (eg, Penicillin Grünenthal)	9.7	15–30	80	40	430	0.1–0.2	
Betamethasone (eg, Betnesol)	5.6±0.8	72	5	35	210±65	1.4±0.3	
Betaxolol	14–22	85	15	45	265–500	7.7–8.8	Slower climination in the elderly
Bezafibrate (Cedur)	1.5–2.1	95	50	5	100–140	0.24	
Bezitramide (Burgodin)	11–24		0.3				
Bifonazole	1–2				35	0.7	
Biperiden (Akineton)	18				146		
Bleomycin (Bleomycinum Mack)	3–9.5		50–70		80–120	0.3–1.7	
Bopindolol	4.18±0.38				515±70.5	2.52±0.37	
Bretylium (eg, Bretilan)	9–14	23±9	80–100	95	300–700	3.4–5.9	
Bromazepam (Lexotanil)	8–22	95	2.3	30	30–100	0.5–2.0	$t_{1/2}$ ↑ in the elderly
Bromhexine (Bisolvon)	15	20		1	800	5.7	
Bromocriptine (Pravidel)	48	>95	<5				

3 Tables with pharmacokinetic data (continued)

Substance (trade name)	$t_{1/2}$ h	F %	A_e^∞ %	f_u %	CL ml/min	V 1/kg	Remarks
Brompheniramine (eg, Dimegan)	25±9.3	80	5			11.7	
Brotizolam (Lendormin)	5	70	<3	7	110	0.7	Delayed elimination in elderly subjects and cirrhosis
Budesonid (Pulmicort)	2.66 2.71	10.7 (oral) 73 (Inhalation)			1946 1111	5.86 3.37	22 R-Enantiomer 22 S-Enantiomer
Buflomedil (Bufedil)	2–4	72	24		362	1.3±0.3	
Bumetanide (Fordiuran)	1.1±0.1	90	66±3	7.4	130±10	0.14±0.01	
Bunitrolol (Stresson)	2	13–40	10		Hepatic		
Buprenorphine (Temgesic)	3.1±0.6	40–90 (i.m.) 100 (subl.)	<5	4	1270±90	2.7±0.5	
Bupivacaine (eg, Carbostesin)	1.3		4–10	10	Hepatic		
Busereline (Suprefact)	1.3	100 (s.c.)					
Buspirone (Bespar)	2–3	39	<1	5	1900	5.3	First pass metabolism to active metabolites

Busulfan (Myleran)	2.6±0.5		1		310±60	1.0±0.2	
Butabarbital (Neravan)	34–42	1	8	74	18	0.8	
Camazepam (Albego)	20–24	100			Hepatic		Temazepam represents active main metabolite
Captopril (Lopirin)	1–2	65	38–50	70	930	0.7	
Carbamazepine (eg, Tegretal)	27±4 15±5	70–80	1–2	20	41±9 90±40	1.4±0.2	Following single dose Following repeated administration (induction!)
Carbamazepine-10,11-Epoxide	6.1±0.7	90	<1	50	100±30	0.7±0.1	
Carbenicillin (eg, Anabactyl)	1.0±0.2		82–99	50	130	0.18	
Carbenoxolone (eg, Biogastrone)	13–26	80	10	0.5	190–280	0.1	Elimination rate decreased in elderly subjects
Carbimazole (eg, Carbimazol-Henning)	6–8		10				$t_{1/2}$ refers to main metabolite thiamazole
Carbutamide (eg. Invenol)	8–89	95	50	45			
Carbuterol (Pirem)	3–4		80	80			

3 Tables with pharmacokinetic data (continued)

Substance (trade name)	$t_{1/2}$ h	F %	A_e^∞ %	f_u %	CL ml/min	V 1/kg	Remarks
Carisoprodol (Sanoma)	8	1	<1	45		0.6	
Carmustine (Carmubris)	1.5				3920	3.3	$t_{1/2}$ of active metabolites 34 h
Carprofen (Imadyl)	13–20	90	5	<1	28±4	0.3	
Cefacetril	0.7–1.3		75	30	360	0.25–0.37	
Cefaclor (Panoral)	0.75	90	60	60		0.24	
Cefadroxil (Bidocel)	1.4±0.2	80–90	>90	90	180	0.24	
Cefalexine (eg, Oracel)	0.9±0.2	90±9	96	84	300±80	0.26±0.03	
Cefaloridin	0.8–1.8		90	80	168	0.22	
Cefalotin (eg, Cephalotin Lilly)	0.6±0.3		52	29	470±120	0.26±0.11	$t_{1/2}$=2 h in newborns
Cefanone	2.5		95	12	54	0.17	
Cefapirin	1.2±0.3		48±7	38	300±110	0.13±0.05	
Cefamandol (Mandokel)	0.8±0.1	95	96±3	26	200±70	0.16±0.05	

Cefazedone (Refosporin)	1.5–2.0		70	6	90	0.14	
Cefazolin (eg. Gramaxin)	1.8±0.4		80±16	16	70±15	0.12±0.03	
Cefmetazole	0.7–1.4		>90		144	0.12	
Cefonicid			88±6	2	23±17	0.1±0.01	
Cefoperazone (Cefobis)	2.1±0.3	100 (i.m.)	25–30	10	20–80	0.1–0.18	About 75% excreted in bile
Ceforanide	2.6±0.5		84±3	20	30	0.14±0.04	
Cefotaxime (Claforan)	1.1±0.2		60–80	30	215±14	0.23±0.01	
Cefotetan	3.1–4.2			15	29.2–49.0	0.11–0.17	
Cefoxitin (Mefoxitin)	0.7±0.1		78	27	400	0.16–0.31	
Cefradin (Sefril)	0.8±0.3	>90	86±10	86	360±85	0.25±0.01	
Cefroxadine	1.0±0.1	>90	95	>90	355±58	0.22	
Cefsulodin (Pseudocel)	1.6±0.2		60	85	140±23	0.43±0.1	
Ceftazidime (Fortum)	1.5–2.8		100	85	72–141	0.2–0.27	
Ceftezole	0.9		87	14		0.12	

3 Tables with pharmacokinetic data (continued)

Substance (trade name)	$t_{1/2}$ h	F %	A_e^∞ %	f_u %	CL ml/min	V 1/kg	Remarks
Ceftizoxime (Ceftix)	0.7–1.4		70–100	72	111–200	0.2–0.38	Clearance is dependent on urinary flow
Ceftriaxone (Recephin)	8±1.3		33–67	4–17	9.7–13	0.11±0.08	fu and CL are concentration dependent
Cefuroxime (Zinacel)	1–2		90–100	67	150	0.2	
Chloralhydrate (Chloraldurat)	8	0	<1	60		0.6	Presystemic elimination to active trichloroethanol, its $t_{1/2}$ is 6–10 h
Chlorambucil (Leukeran)	1.0±0.3	75–100			40±25	0.86±0.81	Active metabolite phenylacetic acid mustard $t_{1/2}=2.5$ h
Chloramphenicol (eg, Leukomycin)	2–5	75–90	25±15	47	260±120	0.94±0.06	Impaired elimination in cirrhosis
Chlordiazepoxide (eg, Librium)	9–18	100	<1	4	20–35	0.25–0.5	In cirrhosis and elderly subjects reduced elimination, active metabolites
Chlormethiazole (Distraneurin)	2.6–4.7				850–1440	2–3.5	
Chloroguanide	15	1	40	30		19.2	
Chloroquine (Resochin)	3.1±2.6 43±7 312±99	>90	50–70	40	Non-lin. kinetics	185±66	Dose: 250 mg Dose: 500 mg Dose: 1 g

Chlorothiazide	1.5 ± 0.2	56 (50 mg) 9 (1 g)	92 ± 5	5	320 ± 120	0.2 ± 0.1	
Chlorphenamine (Polaronil)	20–30	25–60	20–40	28	115–125	3–3.4	
Chlorphenesine (Soorphenesin)	3	1	< 1			1.3	
Chlorpromazine (Megaphen)	10–60	20–60	< 1	4	640	10–35	Hepatic first pass effect to active metabolites
Chlorpropamide (eg, Cloronase)	30–48	> 90	20 ± 18	12	3.3 ± 0.2	0.1 ± 0.1	
Chlortalidone (eg, Hygroton)	44 ± 10	64 ± 10	65 ± 9	25	115 ± 30	3.9 ± 0.8	Renal CL and Ae ↓ in doses higher than 200 mg
Chlortetracycline (Aureomycin)	5–9		< 20	45	32*	1.2	* Renal clearance
Cibenzoline	7.7				632 ± 72	5.8 ± 0.8	
Cimetidine (Tagamet)	2–3	62 ± 6	62 ± 20	81	570 ± 125	1–2	CL ↓ in aged and renal failure
Cinoxacin (Cinobactin)	1.5–2.1		40–60	45	180	0.34	
Ciprofloxacin	3.7 ± 0.9	70–80	45 p.o. 62 i.v.	70–80	994 ± 358	4.31 ± 1.64	
Cisplatin (Platinex)	0.64				1250	0.51	For total platinum ≥ 24 h
Clavulanic acid	0.6–2.5		75	80	174–30	0.1–0.2	

3 Tables with pharmacokinetic data (continued)

Substance (trade name)	$t_{1/2}$ h	F %	A_e^{∞} %	f_u %	CL ml/min	V 1/kg	Remarks
Clenbuterol (Spiropent)	34		36.6	50	60	4	
Clindamycin (Sobelin)	2.7±0.4	87	9–14	6	250±60	0.66±0.1	
Clobazam (Frisium)	25±7	90	<10	12	40	1.4	Active metabolite desmethylclobazam accumulates following multiple administration ($t_{1/2}$ is 36–46 h)
Clofibrate (eg, Regelan)	13±3	95±10	6–15	3.5	13±2	0.11±0.02	
Clonazepam (Rivotril)	20–36	95	<1	18	65±20	3.2±1.1	
Clonidine (eg. Catapresan)	8.5±2.0	75±4	62±11	80	220±85	2.1±0.4	
Clorazepate (Tranxilium)	50–75	100	<1	2	10–17	0.6–1.7	Is a prodrug with $t_{1/2}$=2 h converted to desmethyldiazepam (see these data)
Clotiazepam (Trecalmo)	6		<3	1	220	2.0	Partly active metabolites V↑ in elderly subjects
Clotrimazole (Canesten)	4–6			2			High first pass effect
Cloxacillin (Staphobristol)	0.55±0.1	43±16	75±14	5	155±30	0.1±0.02	

Cocaine	0.7±0.3				2600±650	2.1±1.2	
Codeine (eg, Codicept)	3–4		<10	>90	850±60	3.5±0.2	
Caffeine	4.9±1.8	1.1±0.5	64	100± 40	0.61±0.02		
Colchicine (Colchicum-Dispert)	1.1±0.3				600±155	0.7±0.13	Hepatic elimination
Collistine	3	100 (i.m.)	80	80		0.55	
Convallotoxin	12–19	5		70			
Coumarine	0.8	4	<1	65		1.7	
Cotrimoxazole (eg, Bactrim)	s. Trimetoprim and s. Sulfamethoxazol						
Cyclobarbital (Phanodorm)	8–17				34	0.47	
Cyclophosphamide (eg, Endoxan)	6–10	75	5–25	45–85	60–100	0.75±0.35	
Cyclosporin A (Sandimmun)	16±8	34±11	<1	4	695±75	3.5±2.7	Kinetic parameters from blood concentrations
Cytarabine (eg, Udicil)	2.6±0.6	20	11±8	87	950±280	3.0±1.9	
Dacarbazine (DTIC-Dome)	5		70	95			
Dapsone	28±3	90	15	27	45±13	1.5±0.5	

3 Tables with pharmacokinetic data (continued)

Substance (trade name)	$t_{1/2}$ h	F %	A_e^∞ %	f_u %	CL ml/min	V 1/kg	Remarks
Delorazepam	83						$t_{1/2}$ ↑ in the elderly
Demeclocycline (Ledermycin)	10–15		>20	10–40		1.25	
Desipramine (Petrofran)	18±6	51–68	3±4	10	1700±850	34±8	Non-linear kinetics
Deslanoside (Cedilanid)	44	80	60	3		4.4	
Desmethyldiazepam	50–75	100	<1	2	10–17	0.6–1.7	In elderly and cirrhotic patients delayed elimination
Dexamethasone (eg, Fortecortin)	3	78	3	32	300–500	1	
Dextran (eg, Macrodex)	1.9 3–4 6–8				Renal elimination		Dextran 1 Dextran 40 Dextran 60
Dextromethorphan (Arpha)	2–4	75	20			1.1	
Dextrothyroxine (eg, Dynothel)	6–7 days!	50		<1		0.2	
Diazepam (eg, Valium)	24–48	100 85 (i.m.)	<1	3	20–40	1.1	Accumulation of active metabolites, impaired elimination in cirrhosis, in the elderly $t_{1/2}$ and V ↑

Diazoxide (eg, Hypertonalum)	20–48	86–96	20–50	10	4.5	0.21	
Dibecacin	1.5–2.2		85	>85		0.2–0.3	
Diclofenac (Voltaren)	1.5	60	1	0.8	263±56	0.12±0.04	
Dicloxacillin (Dichlor-Stapenor)	0.7±0.1	50 – 85	60±7	4	115±25	0.09±0.002	Renal clearance in doses above 1–2 g is probably saturated
Diflunisal (Dolobid)	7–11		<10	1.5	8	0.11	Non-linear kinetics
Digitoxin (eg, Digimerck)	5–8	>90	32±15	3	3.5±2	0.54±0.14	
Digoxin (eg, Lanicor)	42±19	75±11	60±11	75	188±44	8.4±2.3	
Dihydroergotamine (eg, Dihydergot)	2.4±0.3	<1	11	7	1000±170	14.5±3.1	Marked presystemic elimination
Diltiazem (Dilzem)	3.1±1.0	42±18	<4	22	1495±560	3–6	
Diphenhydramine (eg, Dolestan)	4–8	40–55	<2	20	850±100	4–7	Following i.v. admin. $t_{1/2}=9.3\pm 0.7$ h after 8 to 12 h
Diphenoxylate	2.5				1.5	3.8	
Dipyramidol (eg, Persantin)	11.6±2.2	43±13		1	138±30	2.0±0.7	
Disopyramide (eg, Norpace)	6–8	83±11	55±6	32–72	90±50	0.6±0.8	f_u concentration dependent

3 Tables with pharmacokinetic data (continued)

Substance (trade name)	$t_{1/2}$ h	F %	A_e^∞ %	f_u %	CL ml/min	V 1/kg	Remarks
Disulfiram (Antabus)	4.8	90	50	50		23	
Dobutamine (Dobutrex)	2.4±0.7 min!				4420±1550	0.2±0.1	
Dopamine	0.15	0	3			0.93	
Domperidone (Motilium)	7.5	15	<1	8	700	5.7	High first pass effect
Dosulepin (Idom)	14–40	65			1020–2100	20–92	Hepatic first pass effect
Doxepin (Eg, Aponal)	17±6	27±10	<1		980±210	20±8	High first pass metabolism to active desmethyldoxepin ($t_{1/2}$ is 33–80 h)
Doxorubicin (Adriblastin)	36±11		<15	20	1250±220	52	
Doxycycline (eg, Vibramycin)	12–24	93	40±20	12	40±13	0.8±0.3	
Droperidol (Dehydrobenzperidol)	2–2.5		<1	13		1.75	
Edrophonium	1.8±0.6				720±190	1.1±0.2	
Enalapril (eg, Xanet)	11	61		>50			

Encainide	3.38±1.68	42		30	957	2.7	Genetic defect in 6 to 10% patients for conversion to active O-desmethyl encainide
Ephedrine (Ephetonin)	4–10	88	55		230–660	1.7–4.3	
Ergotamine (eg, Ergotamin Medihaler)	1.9±0.3	40–60	4		770	1.85	
Erythromycin (Erythrocin)	1.1–3.5	35±25	12±7	25	420–650	0.7–1.6	
Estazolam	14		<4				
Estramustinphosphate (Estracyt)	13.6	44±5	<1		77.0±6.2	0.11	
Ethacrynic acid (Hydromedin)	2–4		66				
Ethambutol (Myambutol)	3.1±0.4	77±8	79±3	75	600±60	1.6±0.2	
Ethionamide	2.1			70			
Ethosuximide (eg, Suxinutin)	45±8 33±6		25±15	100	14±3	0.72±0.16	Adults Children
Etilefrin (eg, Effortil)	2.2±0.2	55	28±3	77	954±13	2.3±0.2	High presystemic elimination
Etomidate (Hypnomidate)	3.9±1.1		<2	23	954±178	4.6±2.2	

3 Tables with pharmacokinetic data (continued)

Substance (trade name)	$t_{1/2}$ h	F %	A_e^{∞} %	f_u %	CL ml/min	V 1/kg	Remarks
Etoposide (Vepesid)	11.5	50	50	84		20	
Etretinate (Tigason)	80–100 days!			<1			
Enprophylline	1.7±0.2		82		353±68	0.65±0.13	
Ethinylestradiol (Progynon M)	3–12	42					Enterohepatic circulation
Famotidine (Pepdul)	2–4	20–66	70	>85	310±11	1.1±0.1	
Felodipine	14	15		<1	1091	9.7	
Fenbufen (Lederfen)	7–14		<10	<1			
Fenfluramine (Ponderax)	18–20	65	40	60		14	
Fenoprofen (Feprona)	2.5–3	>85	<2	<1		0.08–0.11	Renal CL = 39–48 ml/min
Fenoterol (eg, Partusisten)	7	60	<2	60		1.5	
Fenoximon	60±14 i.v. 78±26 oral	53	<1	<1	2062±847	0.37±0.26	

Fentanyl (Fentanyl Janssen)	3.5		8	20	785±240	3.6	
Flecainide (Tambocor)	13.8±2.9	95	42	55	739±275	8.4	Genetic polymorphism
Fluoride (eg, Zymafluor)	1.6–2.7 4.8–6.7	100	38–51		106–224	1	3 mg 10 mg
Flucloxacillin (Staphylex)	0.5–1	50	40–45	5	123±13	0.12±0.02	$t_{1/2}$ dose dependent
Flucytosine (Ancotil)	4.2±0.3	84±6	99±7	96		0.68±0.04	CL ≙ creatinine clearance
Flufenamic acid (Sastridex)	9		20	10		0.1	
Flumazenil (Anexate)	0.7–1.3	15–25	<1	60	520–1300	0.6–1.6	
Flunarizine (Sibelium)	18 days!			0.8	301–443	43.2	
Flunitrazepam (Rohypnol)	15±5	85	<1	20	245	2.5	Active metabolite with $t_{1/2}$ = 20–30 h
Fluocortolone (eg, Ultralan)	1.3±0.3	83–95		12	454±145	1.0±0.3	
Fluorouracil (eg, Fluroblastin)	0.2–0.4	28–58	1–4	90	800–1700	0.2±0.1	$t_{1/2}$ and CL dose dependent, capacity limited first pass effect
Fluoresceine	3	56	64		170	0.53	

3 Tables with pharmacokinetic data (continued)

Substance (trade name)	$t_{1/2}$ h	F %	A_e^∞ %	f_u %	CL ml/min	V 1/kg	Remarks
Fluoxetine	3.6±2.9 days!			5.5	93.9–703.5		
Fluphenazine (eg, Lyogen)	10–18 3.7 days! 6.8–9.6 days!	10–30	<1	1		25	Considerable first pass effect Fluphenazine-enantate (i.m.) Fluphenazine-decanoate (i.m.)
Flupirtine	8.5	90	15		113	1.15	
Flurazepam (Dalmadorm)	2 74±24	30–60	<1 <1	85 3.5	335±165	22±17	High first pass effect to desalkyl flurazepam (this line) and hydroxy ethylflurazepam ($t_{1/2}$=2–10 h)
Flurbiprofen (Froben)	4		25	<1		0.1	
Fosfomycin (Fosfocin)	2		90	>99	132±54	0.21–0.35	
Furazlocillin	0.9±0.2		33±4	30–40	192–480	0.13–0.22	
Furosemide (eg, Lasix)	0.8–1.5	62	70	3	160	0.11	
Fusidic acid (Fucidine)	5.6±1.8	70–100	<5		50	0.16±0.06	
Gallamine	2.2		86		85±22	0.2±0.1	

Gentamicin (eg, Refobacin)	2–3	90 (i.m.)	>90	>90	95	0.25	terminal $t_{1/2} = 53 \pm 25$ h
Gitoformate (Dynocard)	220	85–90		86	3.7		f_u valid for gitoxin
Glibenclamide (Euglucon)	10	40–100	<1	<1		0.1	
Glibornuride (eg, Glutril)	5–11	95	<1	5		0.26	Hepatic elimination
Gliclazide (Nordialex)	6–14		<20	10		0.3	
Glipizide (Glibenese)	2.7–4	>90	<1	4	52 ± 50	0.16	
Glisoxepide (Pro-Diaban)	1.7 ± 0.4	>90	50	7		0.1	
Glutethimide (Doriden)	6–22	<10	<2	46			Active, partly toxic metabolites
Glymidine (Redul)	4	>90	1	8			Active metabolites
Griseofulvine (eg, Flucin)	9–21	30–70	<1	20		15	
Guanethidine (Ismelin)	35–48	20–40	50–60				Terminal $t_{1/2} = 4.8$ days, renal CL 42–91 ml/min

3 Tables with pharmacokinetic data (continued)

Substance (trade name)	$t_{1/2}$ h	F %	A_e^∞ %	f_u %	CL ml/min	V l/kg	Remarks
Guanfacine (Estulic Wander)	18–21	100	30	36	188	3.95	
Haloperidol (eg, Haldol Janssen)	10–24	70±18	<1	8	880±210	18±6.5	
Heparin (eg, Liquemin)	1–2.5		20	10	20–25	0.06±0.01	$t_{1/2}$ and CL are dose dependent
Heptabarbital (Medomin)	6–11		<1		140	1.2	
Hetacillin	1.3		90	80		0.4	
Hexobarbital (Evipan)	3–5	40–60	<1	53	255±60	1.2±0.3	
Hydralazine (eg, Nepresol)	2.2±0.4 2.6±0.4	31±7 50±7	12±0.4 14±0.1	13 13	700±420 560±140	1.6±0.3	Rapid acetylators Slow acetylators
Hydrochlorothiazide (eg, Esidrix)	2.5±0.2	71±15	>95	36	350±80	0.8±0.3	
Hydrocortisone (eg, Ficortril)	1.5	100	<1	5–25	210–295	0.3–0.1	f_u dose dependent
Hydroflumethiazide	11–27	52	47	25		6.4	
Hydromorphone (Dilaudid)	2.6±0.9	62±33	6		400±170	1.2±0.2	Elimination as conjugate

Hydroxychloroquine (Quensyl)	5–7 days!		52	50			
Hydroxyzine (eg, Atarax)	20±4				650±215	16±3	$t_{1/2}$=7.1±2.3 h in children
Ibuprofen (eg, Brufen)	2±0.5	>80	<1	<1	55±15	0.15	Non-linear kinetics through capacity limited protein binding
Ifosfamide (Holoxan)	15.2±3.6		53		30–50	0.86	
Imipramine (Tofranil)	10–24	25–60	<2	6	1400±700	10–30	First pass metabolism to active desipramine
Indamide (Natrilex)	14–16	>90	<10		20±5	25±6	
Indomethacin (eg, Amuno)	2.5–11	98	15±8	10	140±30	0.3–0.9	
Indoramine (Wydora)	5.1±1.0	8					$t_{1/2}$ age dependent
Insulin	1.5–2	0	5	95		0.6	
Isoconazole (Travogen)	27	10					
Isoflurane (Forene)	3.8					49±33	
Isoniazid (eg, Neoteben)	1.1±0.2 3.0±0.8		7±2 29±5	 100	490 175	0.6±0.1	Rapid acetylators Slow acetylators

3 Tables with pharmacokinetic data (continued)

Substance (trade name)	$t_{1/2}$ h	F %	A_e^∞ %	f_u %	CL ml/min	V 1/kg	Remarks
Isosorbiddinitrate (eg, Isoket)	0.5–1.5	22±14 (p.o.) 59±29 (subl.) 33±17 (perc.)	1	72	1750	1.8	Variable first pass metabolism to active mononitrates
Isosorbide-2-mononitrate	1.9±0.5	100			430±115	0.8±0.3	
Isosorbide-5-mononitrate (eg, Elantan)	4.4±0.5	93±13	<5	100	135±20	0.8±0.1	
Isotretinoin (Roaccutan)	17–20	60		0.1	134–202	0.95	
Isoxicam (Pacyl)	20–40	70		3	6	0.2	Bioavailability increases when administered with meal by about 25%
Josamycin (Wilprafen)	1.7±0.4		5	15		3.3–11.8	
Kanamycin (eg, Kanamytrex)	2.1±0.2		90	100	100±15	0.26±0.05	
Ketamine (Ketanest)	3.6±1.4	20±7	2.3±0.5	>95	1350±180	2.9±0.7	
Ketanserine	12.6±4.8	27–69	<4	6	410±62	6.2±1.5	
Ketazolam (Contamix)	1.5		<1	7			Very rapid metabolism to active diazepam and desmethyldiazepam

Ketobemidone (Cliradon)	3.9±1.7	34	6		1260±300	5.9±2.6	
Ketoconazole (Nizoral)	6.5–9	75	2–4	1		0.36	
Ketoprofen (eg, Orudis)	2	>90	<1	1.5	106±38	0.1±0.02	
Labetalol (Trandate)	5.2±1.3	25	<5	50	1650±630	10±2	
Laevomethadone (L-Polamidon)	35±12	92	25	11	100±35	3.8±0.6	
Lamoxactam/Latamoxef (Moxalactam)	1–4		80	60	84±12	0.3	
Lanatosid (eg, Cedilanid)	40	20–60	15 (p.o.) 70 (i.v.)	80		4.4	Following oral administration, partly converted to digoxin in gastrointestinal tract
Levodopa (eg, Lavodopa)	0.44	90	<1	95		12.7	
Levomepromazine (Neurocil)	17–78				530–6590		Presystemic sulfoxidation
Levothyroxine (eg, Euthyrox)	6–7 days!	70	<1	0.5	0.83	0.1–0.2	
Levorphanol	11	50–100			60±2.6		
Lidocaine (eg, Xylocain)	1.8±0.4	35±11	2±1	30	650±170	1.1±0.4	CL ↓ if the infusion ≥ 24 h

3 Tables with pharmacokinetic data (continued)

Substance (trade name)	$t_{1/2}$ h	F %	A_e^∞ %	f_u %	CL ml/min	V 1/kg	Remarks
Lincomycin (eg, Albiotic)	4–7		10	20–30	78	0.4–0.2	
Lithium (eg, Lithium-Duriles)	22±8	100	95±15	100	25±8	0.8±0.3	
Lofepramine (Gamonil)	4.7			1			
Lonazolac (eg, Argun)	6	63–85		1–8		1.5	
Loperamide (Imodium)	7–15	Low	1–2	4	Hepatic		Marked first pass effect
Loprazolam (eg, Dormonoct)	7–10		<1	20	510±30	4.0±0.5	
Lorazepam (Tavor)	14±5	93±10	<1	7	80±30	1.3±0.2	
Lorcainide (Remivox)	7.7±2.2	30–100	<2	17±3	1002±304	7.8±2.9	F dose dependent, capacity limited first pass effect
Lormetazepam (Noctamid)	10.6±2.4	80	<20	<15	230±60	4.6	
Maprotiline (Ludiomil)	58±29	79–84	2		233	14.3	
Marcellomycin	20–50		<8		1550		

Mebendazole (Vermox)	1.2	17	<10	5		2.0	
Medazepam (Nobrium)	2	49–76	1	0.2			Marked first pass metabolism to active metabolites with $t_{1/2}=30-100$ h
Mefanamic acid (eg, Parkemed)	2			1			
Mefruside (Baycaron)	3–12		0.5		375–2150	4.5–7.4	
Melperone (Eunerpan)	3–8	64±17	5–10		2190±700	7.0±1.6	
Melphalan (Alkeran)	1.4±0.2	71±23	12±7		390±200	0.6±0.2	
Mepindolol (Corindolan)	4			40–60		5.7	
Mepivacaine (Scandicain)	2–3		1	30			
Meptazinole (Meptid)	1.9±0.1		<5	66.2	1373	5.0	
Meprobamate (eg, Cyrpon)	12.6±2.5	90	10	100		0.7	$t_{1/2}=24.3\pm4.4$ h in chronic liver diseases
Meproscillarin (Cliff)	50	60–70	20	10			
Mercaptopurine (Puri-Nethol)	0.9±0.4	12±7	22±12	81	820±300	0.56±0.38	F=60% if first pass metabolism by allopurinol is inhibited

3 Tables with pharmacokinetic data (continued)

Substance (trade name)	$t_{1/2}$ h	F %	A_e^{∞} %	f_u %	CL ml/min	V 1/kg	Remarks
Mesalazine (eg, Salofalk)	0.7–2.4	10–45* (absorbed amount)	10–15	57	300±67	0.26±0.1	* Depending on dosage form
Mesuximide (Petinutin)	2.6		1				Demethylated active metabolite ($t_{1/2}$ = 38 h)
Metaclazepam (Talis)	18–20		<1		520		
Metacycline	9–15		>20	20–25		1.6	
Metamizole (s. Noramidopyrinmethane sulfonate)							
Metformine (Glucophage retard)	1.7±0.1	50–60	100	100	454±47	1.0±0.06	$t_{1/2}$ determined through absorption rate following p.o. administration
Methamphetamine (Pervitin)	5–6			80		3.5–4.6	$t_{1/2}$ increases (20–30 h) if the urine is alkaline
Methapyrilen	1.1–2.1	4–46	<2		910–3360	2.1–6.6	
Methaqualone (eg, Revonal)	20–40	>90	2	15		6	
Methenamine (eg, Aci-steril)	20	80	90			0.6	

Methicillin (Cinopenil	0.9±0.2		88±17	60	430±90	0.43±0.1	
Methohexital (Brevimytal)	3.9±2.1		<1	20	810±220	2.2±0.7	
Methotrexate (eg, Methotrexate Lederle)	5.3 children 7.4 adults	65	85±11	50	110±25	0.9±0.2	$t_{1/2}$ is concentration dependent
Methyldopa (eg, Presinol)	1.8±0.2	25±16	28±9	90	220±65	0.4±0.1	
Methylphenobarbital (Prominal)	50	73	1–2		40	2.44	Partly metabolised to phenobarbital
Methylprednisolone (eg, Urbason)	2.5±0.8	82±13	5	50	280±65	0.8±0.2	
Metildigoxin (Lanitop)	40–70	70–90	70	25	125±40	6.2±1.6	
Metoclopramide (eg, Paspertin)	3.6–5.3	53 (supp.) 79 (drops)	20	>90	640±140	3.1±0.6	
Metoprolol (eg, Beloc)	3.2±0.2	38±14	10±3	87	1050±210	4.2±0.7	
Metronidazole (Clont)	6–14	99±8 80 (supp.)	<10	90	50–100	0.6–1.1	
Mexiletine (Mexitil)	8–18	87±13	8–15 50 (pH 5.0)	37	350–770	5–10	
Mezlocillin (Baypen)	0.7–1.3		8–36	70	200–325	0.15–0.3	Ae, CL and V are dose dependent

3 Tables with pharmacokinetic data (continued)

Substance (trade name)	$t_{1/2}$ h	F %	A_e^∞ %	f_u %	CL ml/min	V 1/kg	Remarks
Mianserine (Tolvin)	8–19	30	5	10	79±43	13.8±7.8	
Miconazole (Daktar)	20–24	27	1	8		21	
Midazolam (Dormicum)	1.5–3	44±17	<1	3	250–600	0.7±0.2	Hepatic first pass effect
Minocycline (Klinomycin)	18±4	100	11±2	24	20±10	0.4±0.1	
Minoxidile (Lonolox)	3.1±0.6	95	12	>95	11	12±3	
Misonidazole	9.4±0.5 10.7±0.5				47.4±3.2 40.9±2.8	0.54±0.05 0.52±0.05	(+)-Enantiomer (−)-Enantiomer
Mitoxantrone (Novantron)	43±20		6.5	10	980	45	
Molsidomine (Corvaton)	1.6±1.0	44±15			982		
Morphine	3.0±1.2	20–33	8	65	1050±150	3.3±0.9	
Moxalactam	2.1±0.7	85 (i.m.)	76±12	50	130	0.25±1	
Nabilone	2	96			48.3		
N-Acetylcystein (Fluimucil)	2.3±0.3		30		233±20	0.33±0.03	

N-Acetylprocainamide (NAPA)	6.0±0.2	83±12	81±4	90	220±30	1.4±0.2	Active metabolite of procainamide
Nadolol (Solgol)	16±2	34±5	73±4	80	205±45	2.1±1.0	
Nafcillin	1.0±0.2	36	27±5	11	560±135	0.35±0.1	
Nafimidone	2–4		<1			75	Active metabolite (nalimidone alcohol) with $t_{1/2}=3.3$ h
Nalidixic acid (Nogram)	2.7±0.7	90	4	5	140±30	0.5±0.1	
Naloxone (Narcanti)	1.2	20	<1		1820	2.0	Marked first pass metabolism to glucuronide
Naproxene (eg, Proxen)	14±1	95±6	<1	0.1–2.4	9.5±1.5	0.16±0.02	f_u is concentration dependent
Sodiumthiosulfate	1.3±0.63		28.5±9.4		328±131	1.73	
Nefopam (Ajan)	3–8	50	<5	28			
Neomycin (eg, Bykomycin)	2.5	3	50			0.2	
Neostigmine (Prostigmin)	1.3±0.8	2	50–67		590±190	0.7±0.3	
Netilmicin (Certomycin)	2.3±0.7 37±6		85	>90	95±15	0.21±0.03	 Terminal $t_{1/2}$
Nicardipine	4.8±3.1				596.6±195	20.6±6.3	

3 Tables with pharmacokinetic data (continued)

Substance (trade name)	$t_{1/2}$ h	F %	A_e^∞ %	f_u %	CL ml/min	V 1/kg	Remarks
Nicotine (Nicorette chewing gum)	2.0±0.7		2–25	95	1350±390	2.6±0.9	Ae is pH dependent
Nicotinic acid (Niconacid)	0.3–0.8	88	35				
Nifedipine (Adalat)	3.4±1.2	45±28	<1	2	750±375	1.2±0.5	
Nifenazone (Nicopyron)	8–24		40–90				
Niflumic acid (Actol)	2.5			15	45	0.12	
Nitrazepam (eg, Mogadan)	29±7	78±16	<1	14	70±35	2.4±0.8	
Nitrendipine (Bayotensin)	8	20	<1	2	1400	5.4±2.4	High first pass effect
Nitrofurantoin (Furadantin)	1±0.3	90	47±13	40	250±55	0.6±0.1	
Nitroglycerine (eg, Nitrolingual)	2.3±0.6 min.!	38±26	<1		16000±6300	3.3±1.2	Very marked presystemic elimination to active metabolites
Nizatidine	1.3±0.23				790±250	1.21±0.51	
Nomifensine (Alival)	2–5		63	40	175–300	5.4–8.4	

Noramidopyrinmethane-sulfonate Metamizole (eg, Novalgin)	6.9±1.0	>90	<2			
Norepinephrine (Arterenol)	1–2 min!	3	4–16	50		
Norfenefrine (eg, Novadral)	3	20	3			
Norfloxacine (Barazan)	2.2–4.5		24–36	>85		
Nortriptyline (Nortrilen)	31±13	51±5	2	8	525±130	18±4
Noscapine (Capval)	2.6±0.5	30±7			1540±190	4.7±0.9
Ofloxacine (Tarivid)	6	90	94	97	241±54	2.5±0.8
Orciprenaline (Alupent)	1.5	33		90		
Ornidazole (Tiberal)	13	90		>85	82	1.0
Oxacillin (eg, Stapenor)	0.4–0.7	33	46	8	445±125	0.33±0.1
Oxatomide (Tinset)	14		<1	2		
Oxazepam (eg, Adumbran)	8–15	80	<2	10	90–140	1.0

3 Tables with pharmacokinetic data (continued)

Substance (trade name)	$t_{1/2}$ h	F %	A_e^∞ %	f_u %	CL ml/min	V 1/kg	Remarks
Oxazolam (Tranquit)	1.5		<1				Very rapid metabolism to active desmethyldiazepam
Oxmetidine	2.7	30–90	<5		150–210	0.6±0.2	
Oxolinic acid (Nidantin)	4 (15)		5	20			
Oxprenolol (Trasicor)	2.3	25–60	<5	20	400	1.2	F variable because of first pass effect
Oxyphenbutazone (eg, Tanderil)	27–64	>90	<2	1		0.14	Active metabolite of phenylbutazone
Oxytetracycline (Terramycin)	10	60–80	70	75		1.5	
Pancuronium (Pancuronium "Organon")	1.5–2.5		67±18	80	130±30	0.2±0.1	
Papaverine (eg, Panergon)	1.8	26	<1	7	740	0.58	
Paracetamol (Eg, Ben-u-ron)	2.0±0.4	89±10	3	85	350±100	0.95±0.13	In overdoses (due to liver damage) $t_{1/2}$ upto 12 h prolonged
Pefloxacine	11±3				156	1.9±0.3	
Pemoline (Tradon)	11.0±1.2		47±8	50	52±20	0.65	

Penbutolol (Betapressin)	26	100	10	<5		0.3	
Pengitoxin (Carnacid-Cor)	55–61	70–85		5	12.1	0.95	Active form is 16-acetylgitoxin (Ae=35%, f_u=15%)
Penicillamine (eg, Metalcaptase)	2.5		12		530–2300		
Pentazocine (Fortral)	3.4±1.2	18±8	13	39	1380±320	5.6±1.6	Strong first pass effect
Pentobarbital (Repocal)	20–30	100	1	60	30	0.8	
Pentoxifylline (Trental)	1.4±0.8	20–30	<3	>90	1333±481	2.3±1.1	
Perphenazine (Decentan)	8–12	15–99		1780	10–35		
Peruvoside (Encordin)	40–60			37		11	
Pethidine (Dolantin)	3.2±0.8	52±3	4–22	42	1200±350	4.2±1.3	Ae is pH dependent
Phenacetin	0.7–1.3	20–25	3	65	1440	1–2.1	Capacity limited first pass metabolism to active paracetamol-tamol (s. dort)
Pheneticillin	1.3			12		0.35	
Pheniramine (Avil)	16–19	75	>90		100	1.9	

3 Tables with pharmacokinetic data (continued)

Substance (trade name)	$t_{1/2}$ h	F %	A_e^∞ %	f_u %	CL ml/min	V 1/kg	Remarks
Phenobarbital (eg, Luminal)	75–120	100±11	24±5	49	4.4±0.9	0.54±0.03	Ae is pH dependent
Phenoxymethylpenicillin (eg, Isocillin)	0.5–0.8	30–60	20–30	40		0.73	
Phenprocoumon (Marcumar)	160	>90	<1	1		0.13	
Phenylbutazone (eg, Butazolidin)	30–175	90 55 (supp.)	1	1–3	1.5	0.1–0.15	$t_{1/2}$ and f_u dose/concentration dependent, metabolism to active metabolites
Phenylethylmalonamide (PEMA)	16±3	91±4	79±5	>95	38±8	0.7±0.1	An active metabolite of primidone
Phenytoin (eg, Zentropil)	6–60	98±7	4	10	Hepatic	0.5–0.8	$t_{1/2}$ dose/concentration dependent, non-linear kinetics with $V_{max}=7.5\pm2$ mg/kg/die and $K_m=5.7\pm2.9$ mg/l
Pinacidil	2.1±0.5		6	60	518±160		
Pindolol (eg, Visken)	3.5±0.6	70–90	40–55	49	400–625	2.3±0.9	
Piperacillin (Pipril)	0.9±0.1	70–80 (i.m.)	71±14	50–70	190±50	0.18±0.03	
Pipemidic acid (Deblaston)	0.4		50–70	70–85	384	0.85	

Pirenzepine (Gastrozepin)	10–14	26±5	>80	90	255		
Piretanide (Arelix)	1–1.7		40–75	10	166–250	0.3	
Piroxicam (Felden)	40±5	>90	8	1	2.3–3.5	0.12	
Piroximone	3.2±1.2 2.5±0.3	 81±12	50±5 41±7		661±168 850±223	2.5±0.5 2.6±0.7	i.v. p.o.
Pirprofen (Rengasil)	6	>80	1–5	<1			$t_{1/2}$=40 h in synovial fluid
Polymyxin B	4.4		60				
Polythiazide (Drenusil)	26		25	16		4	
Prajmaliumbitartrate (Neo-Gilurythmal)	2.2±0.6 12.0±0.6	 78	4±3 34±1	39	700±290 82±12	1.4	Normal hydroxylators Deficient hydroxylators
Practolol	5–15	95	90	68		1.6	
Pralidoxime (PAM)	1.1±0.2		85	>90	522±150	0.6±1	
Pramiracetam	5.0				30	2.2	
Prazepam (Demetrin)	1.3±0.7				10000±7000	14.4±5.1	Presystemic elimination to active desmethyldiazepam
Praziquantel (Cesol)	1.5		<1				Marked first pass effect

3 Tables with pharmacokinetic data (continued)

Substance (trade name)	$t_{1/2}$ h	F %	A_e^∞ %	f_u %	CL ml/min	V 1/kg	Remarks
Prazosine (Minipress)	2.9±0.8	57±10	<1	5	210±20	0.6±0.13	
Prednisolone (eg, Decortin-H)	2.1–4.0	82±13	15±5	5–30	100±20	0.5±0.1	$t_{1/2}$ and f_u dose/concentration dependent
Prednisone (eg, Decortin)	3.6±0.4	80±11	3	25	250±60	1.0	
Primaquine (Primaquine Bayer)	6.3±1.4		1		462±77	3.1±0.3	
Primidone (eg, Mylepsinum)	8±5	92±18	42±15	81	70±25	0.6±0.5	Metabolism to active phenylethyl malonamide and phenobarbital
Probenecid (Benemid)	4–12	>95	1–10	10	15–35	0.15	$t_{1/2}$ and CL are dose dependent
Procainamide (eg, Novocamid)	3.0±0.6	83±16	67±8	84	580 420	1.9±0.3	Rapid acetylators Slow acetylators
Prochlorperazine	6.8±0.7				2766±333	21.1±2.2	
Procyclidine (Osnervan)	12				68	1	
Promethazine (Atosil)	12–15	25	<1			10–30	

Propafenone (Rytmonorm)	3–4	49	1	3–13		2–3	f_u concentration dependent, genetic polymorphism
Propanidide (Epontol)				<2	60	Hepatic	Rapid ester hydrolysis to inactive metabolites
Propanthelinbromide (Corrigast)	2.2–3.7	6	17		1320	2.1	
Propicillin (eg, Baycillin)	0.5	50–60		15		0.73	$t_{1/2}\uparrow$ in the elderly, renal failure, newborns
D-Propoxyphene	18	20	<2	24	1060	22.3	
Propranolol (eg, Dociton)	3.9±0.4	36±10	<0.5	7	850±210	3.9±0.4	Capacity limited hepatic first pass effect
Propylthipuracil (Propycil)	0.9–1.4		<10	25	200–370	0.4	
Propyphenazone (in Ozabran)	7–20	>90	10	90			
Proscillaridine (eg, Talusin)	40–50	20–40	<2	15			Partly hydrolysed in stomach
Protriptyline (Maximed)	78±11	77–93		8	255±45	22±1	
Pyridostigmine (Mestinon)	1.9±0.2	14±3	80–90		600±120	1.1±0.3	
Pyrimethamine (Daraprim)	83±14		65	13	30±5	2.9±0.5	
Pyritinol	2.5		<5				

3 Tables with pharmacokinetic data (continued)

Substance (trade name)	$t_{1/2}$ h	F %	A_e^∞ %	f_u %	CL ml/min	V 1/kg	Remarks
Quazepam	39						Active metabolites
Quinidine (eg, Chinidin-Duriles)	6.2±1.8	80 (sulfate) 71 (gluconate)	18±15	10	330±130	2.7±1.2	
Quinine (Chininum sulfuricum Buchler)	11±2			30	140±35	1.8±0.4	
Ranitidine (eg, Zantic)	2–3	50–80	50–70	85	710±62	1.6–2.1	
Reserpine (eg, Sedaraupin)	270	40	<1	60			Marked first pass effect
Ribavirin	36±14	45	35	>99	283±37	8.6±3.4	Accumulation in erythrocytes
Rifampicin (eg, Rifa)	2–4	50–90	5–20	11	620±65	1.6±0.2	Active deacylated metabolite
Rolitetracycline (Reverin)	10	70	60	50		0.6	
Saccharin	5.5–9	100	100	25	287	3.8±1.7	
Salazosulfapyridine (eg, Azulfidine)	5.5±1.2 15.3±2.2	80	<10	50	135±50 37±12	0.9±0.4	rapid and slow acetylation of primary metabolite sulfapyridine,
	0.7–2.4	10–45	10–15	57			active metabolite 5-aminosalicylic acid

Salicylic acid (eg, Guttaplast)	2.4–19	100	2–30	5–20	62±11 14±1 13±2	0.17±0.03	at 11–16 µg/ml at 134–157 µg/ml at 254–312 µg/ml Non-linear kinetics, $t_{1/2}$, f_u, CL dose/concentration dependent, Ae is dependent on urinary pH
Scopolamine	1–4				930±1130	1.1±0.6	
Secobarbital	15–40	90	5		65	1.5	
Sisomicin (eg, Extramycin)	1.9		>90	100	55	0.25	
Sotalol (Sotalex)	6–13	>95	60–75		125±55	1.5±0.5	
Sparteine (Depasan)	2.6		30		535	1.65	6–8% of population are deficient metabolisers
Spectinomycin	1	100	75			0.12	
Spironolactone (eg, Aldactone)	17±3		<1	2			$t_{1/2}$ refers to the active metabolite canrenone
Streptomycin (eg, Streptothenat)	5.3±2.2		39±12	52	30	0.18±0.11	
g-Strophanthine (eg, Purostrophan)	12–40	0.5–4.4	66–90	>95		12–20	For k-strophanthine (cymarine) F should be 15–33%
Sulbactam	1.0±0.1				264±48	0.27–0.4	
Sulbenicillin	0.5–2.0				42–162	0.21	

3 Tables with pharmacokinetic data (continued)

Substance (trade name)	$t_{1/2}$ h	F %	A_e^{∞} %	f_u %	CL ml/min	V 1/kg	Remarks
Sulfadiazine (Sulfadiazin-Heyl)	7.0±3.9	100	62	46	40±12	0.29±0.04	
Sulfamerazine	8–27		12–43			0.24–0.31	
Sulfamethoxazole	10.1±4.6	100	15–30	38	25±3	0.21±0.02	
Sulfametrole	6–12		22			0.16	
Sulfisoxazole (Gantrisin)	6–10	100	50	9	25	0.15–0.4	
Sulfisomidine (Aristamid)	7.5	80	9	14		0.31	
Sulfinpyrazone (Anturano)	4–9	>90	25–50	1.5	20–25	0.1	Partly active metabolites with $t_{1/2}$ upto 14 h
Sulindac (Imbaral)	7	88	<2	4			Renal CL=45±16 ml/min, active metabolite with $t_{1/2}$=18 h
Sulpiride (Dogmatil)	4–7	27±9	70±9		415±84	2.7±0.7	
Tamoxifen (eg, Kessar)	3–21			<1			
Temazepam (eg, Planum)	6–16	>80	<2	2.5	110±50	0.8±0.2	
Temocillin (Temopren)	5.2±0.3			13	18.5±3.2	0.15±0.01	

Terbutaline (eg, Bricanyl)	16±3	15±6	57±14	75	220±35	1.4±0.4	
Testosterone (eg, Testoviron)	0.2–0.3		<1	<3			
Tetracycline (eg, Hostacyclin)	8–12	77	50–60	35	125±20	1.5±0.1	
Tetrazepam (Musaril)	15–22		<1	30	325	3–7	$t_{1/2}$ of active metabolite nortetrazepam in about 36 h
Tetroxoprim	5–9		85–90			0.4–0.8	
Theophylline (eg, Aminophyllin)	9.0±2.1	96±8	8–13	44	50±25	0.50±0.16	
Thiamazole (Favistan)	5.3±0.3		93		96.5±23.8	0.62±0.11	
Thiopental (Trapanal)	8–12		<1	15	230±85	2.1±0.5	
Thioridazine (Melleretten)	4–10 (15–28)					2–6	Active metabolites
Thyroxine	96–168	70	<1	0.05		0.15	
Tiaprofenic acid (Surgam)	1.5–2.5		45	2	100	0.12	
Ticarcillin (Aerugipen)	1.3±0.1		92±2	45	140±15	0.21±0.03	
Tilidine (Valoron N)	3	>90	<10				Contains opiate antagonist (naloxone), active metabolite (nordilidine) with $t_{1/2}=6$ h

3 Tables with pharmacokinetic data (continued)

Substance (trade name)	$t_{1/2}$ h	F %	A_e^∞ %	f_u %	CL ml/min	V 1/kg	Remarks
Timolol (Temserin)	3–5	50–75	15–20	90	540±230	1.9±0.8	
Tinidazole (eg, Simplotan)	12	96	21–33	88	42±8	0.65±0.08	
Tombramycin (eg, Gernebcin)	2.2±0.1 100±57		≥90	90	80	0.26±0.1	Terminal $t_{1/2}$
Tocainide (Xylotocan)	13.5±2.3	89±5	38±7	50	190±35	3.0±0.2	
Tolamolol	2.5	30	5	9		3.1	
Tolazamide (Norglycin)	4.7–8		15				
Tolbutamide (eg, Rastinon)	5.9±1.4	93±10	<1	4	21±4	0.15±0.03	
Tolfenaminic acid	2.5±0.6	60	9	0.3	155±15	0.15±0.03	
Tolmetine (Tolectin)	6.8±1.5	90±11	4–15	1	100±25	10.5±3.0 (1.2±0.6)	
Tomoxetine	4.3±0.5				725±168	3.66±0.79	
Tramadole (Tramal)	6	60–70	<10	95	440	0.31	
Tranexamic acid (eg, Anvitoff)	7	27–35	95		115	0.13	

Tranylcypromine (Parnate)	1.2 1.8		2–6				(+)-Isomer (−)-Isomer Ae pH-dependent
Transdihydrolisuride	2	20–48	0.1	30			f is dose dependent
Trazodone (Thombran)	7–8		1	8			
Triamcinolone (eg, Volon)	>200	90		20			
Triamterene (Jatropur)	2–5	30–65	4	39	980±490	2.5±0.8	Active metabolite with $t_{1/2}=3.1$ h
Triazolam (Halcion)	2–4	55–85	2	15	350–580	0.6–2.3	
Trimazosine	3	63			66		
Trimethadione (Tridione)	16		<5			0.6	Active metabolite dimethadione is slowly eliminated (6% per da)
Trimethoprim (eg, Trimanyl)	11±1.4	100	50–90	30 (60)	155±45	1.8±0.2	
Trimipramine (eg, Stangyl)	23±1.9	41.4±4.4		5.1	1152±108		
TRIS	4–9		>90		95–130	0.7–1.1	
Tubocurarine (Curarin-Asta)	2–4		40–80	50	165±50	0.3±0.1	
Urapidil (Ebrantil)	2.7	72	15				

3 Tables with pharmacokinetic data (continued)

Substance (trade name)	$t_{1/2}$ h	F %	A_e^∞ %	f_u %	CL ml/min	V 1/kg	Remarks
Valproic acid (eg, Orfiril)	8–15	80–100	1.8–2.4	6–20	8.5±3	0.13±0.04	f_u is concentration dependent
Vancomycin (Vancomycin HCl)	5.6±1.8		>90	45	75±5	0.4±0.1	
Veralipride	4		30		250*		*renal CL
Verapamil (eg, Isoptin)	3–8	10–30	<3	10	1200	4.0±1.0	High stereoselective first pass effect
Viloxazine (Vivalan)	2–5	>95	12–15				
Vinblastine (Velbe)	24.8±7.5			10			High affinity for erythrocytes
Vincamine (eg, Cetal)	1.6–2.5	30	6	36		0.58	
Vincristine (Vincristin Lilly)	2.7–3.2		5				60% biliary excretion
Vindesine (Eldisine)	24					8.8	
Vinylbital (Speda)	18–33				30	0.85	
Viomycin	2		80	95		0.24	

Vitamin C = Ascorbic acid (eg, Cebion)	10–16	70–98	>95	76	83	1.2	
Warfarin (Coumadin)	37±5	100	<1	1	3.2±1.7	0.11±0.01	$t_{1/2}$ of R(+)-Enantiomer>(S−)-form CL of R(+)-Enantiomer is about 1/3 of S(−)-form
Xipamide (Aquaphor)	7±1	73			35±4	0.28±0.05	
Zimelidine	4.3–6	30	<1	10		3	
Zomepirac (Zomax)	4 9–16	>90	22	1.5		0.6	 Upon long term therapy
Zopiclone	2–6.5	80	4	55	230	1.3	$t_{1/2}$ abaut 8 h in the elderly and cirrhosis